7 STRATEGIES TO IMPROVE YOUR BOTTOM LINE

The Healthcare Executive's Guide

D0874342

7 STRATEGIES TO IMPROVE YOUR BOTTOM LINE

The Healthcare Executive's Guide

E. PRESTON GEE

Health Administration Press
ACHE Management Series

05   04   03   02   01   5   4   3   2   1

Library of Congress Cataloging-in-Publication Data

7 strategies to improve your bottom line: the healthcare executive's guide / E. Preston Gee.
    p. cm.
    Includes bibliographical references.
    ISBN 1-56793-157-X (alk. paper)
    1. Health services administrators.   2. Health facilities—Business management.   3. Health services administration—Economic aspects. I. Title: Seven strategies to improve your bottom line.   II. Gee, Erin Preston.
    RA971.3.A13   2001
    362.1'068—dc21   2001024610

The paper used in this publication meets the minimum requirements of American National Standard for Information Sciences—Permanence of Paper for Printed Library Materials, ANSI Z39.48-1984.⊗™

Project manager/editor: Joyce Sherman; book designer/cover designer: Matt Avery.

Health Administration Press
A division of the Foundation
    of the American College of
    Healthcare Executives
One North Franklin Street
Suite 1700
Chicago, IL 60606
312/424-2800

Contents

Foreword to 7 *Strategies to Improve Your Bottom Line: The Healthcare Executive's Guide*

AMERICA'S HEALTHCARE SYSTEM is broke, literally and figuratively. Profit margins at the nation's 5,000 acute-care hospitals slipped to 1.8 percent in 1999, the lowest in five years, according to the American Hospital Association. Losses of $200–$300 million have been experienced by some large integrated health systems like Henry Ford and Catholic Healthcare West, and bond ratings have plunged for healthcare provider organizations. Congress responded to the plight of financially ailing hospitals with an $11 billion Medicare relief package in late 2000, but many hospitals are not out of fiscal hot water yet. Pharmaceutical costs rose by 15 percent last year, and a national nursing shortage is driving up wages. If not for investment income, one in four hospitals would not have had a positive bottom line last year. Slumping stock prices on Wall Street are keeping worried hospital administrators awake at night, wondering where they will find the monies to keep the doors open. Fears of closure are rising. *Futurescan 2001*, a national survey of healthcare executives published by Health Administration Press that I authored for the Society of Healthcare Strategy and Market Development, predicts that the number of hospital closings could double, to 50 per year, by 2005.

In the midst of all this financial gloom and doom, a book on how to grow revenues in healthcare organizations could hardly come at a better time. Preston Gee's *7 Strategies to Improve Your Bottom Line* has all the characteristics of a best-seller—a hot topic with managers (money) and a short list of innovative ways to make it (seven).

"This book is not about global solutions, industrywide opportunities, or broad-reaching efforts to save healthcare." Like Stephen Covey's highly popular "7 Habits" series, Preston Gee's advice is simple and direct. The conventional wisdom among hospitals is to grow the medical staff, invest heavily in technology, and build new facilities. Gee's seven strategies, however, do not include any of these widely accepted strategic dictates. Many other industries are being transformed by the Internet and global competition. Not healthcare.

"Recent articles in the trade press have called attention to this disconcerting practice of delaying acceptance of otherwise common business practices." With the collapse of managed care as a constraining force on health costs, Gee recognizes that today, hospitals are competing in a consumer-choice market. With easy access to the Internet, health-seeking consumers— especially the baby boomers—are more informed than any generation of consumers American healthcare has ever treated.

Read the *7 Strategies* and learn something new. "These strategies are not common practice. . . ." Included among the seven strategies are some decidedly unconventional ideas, including streamling (eliminating unprofitable service lines), "co-opetition" (collaborating with competitors), and thinking of the

uninsured as a "market." Most healthcare executives believe
their customers are physicians, managed care plans, and patients. Gee argues that "the two most important customer groups
in the healthcare industry are the government and major employers. . . ." Relating to these big-volume customers takes entirely different market outlooks and tactics.

Preston Gee is one of the best and brightest market analysts in the health industry. He is the author of best-selling anal-
yses of Columbia/HCA and other leading for-profit companies
in healthcare, and he has written frequently during the past 15
years on strategy and management in the health field. This latest
work, *7 Strategies to Improve Your Bottom Line*, is the new unconventional wisdom for healthcare organizations to grow their
markets and boost their bottom lines in the new millennium.

Russell C. Coile, Jr.
National Strategy Advisor
Superior Consultant, Inc.
Southfield, MI
April 14, 2001

Preface

One meets his destiny often in the road he takes to avoid it.

—French proverb

I DECIDED TO write this book a couple of years ago when I witnessed the financial claustrophobia that hospitals and health systems were beginning to encounter. The manuscript took me longer than expected to complete; in that time the economic constraints have become even tighter, the margins thinner, and the outlook bleaker. The time is right and the market is ready for this type of anthology.

As an anthology, the book represents a compilation of concepts and initiatives that I have written about, lectured on, and believed in for several years. For example, chapter one, on streamlining the organization through effective service line management, is nothing original to the industry, nor is it new to me. Jim Folger and I wrote a book on the topic in 1987. At that time, the concept was somewhat fresh and very much on the vanguard for healthcare. Since that time, seminars have been convened, experts have postulated, and consulting firms have profited on the concept. Yet few hospitals or health systems understand the fundamental concept, and fewer still have executed it successfully.

Whereas service line management (we used to call it product line management) may be the patriarch in the family of strategies in this book, it is not likely the one with the greatest potential, nor with the least degree of risk. The other strategies range from the relatively unpracticed ("co-opetition") to the almost-universally misapplied (Internet). Between these are more "fringe options" (retail and visual traffic) and yet-to-be-proven possibilities (complementary and alternative medicine, or CAM). Overall, the seven strategies described represent a portfolio of moderate risk strategies, the main function of which may be to stretch the imagination and challenge the current mode of thinking.

Some might argue, "But there's nothing really *new* in here." I address that argument with two points. First, healthcare executives are not known to try things that *are* really new. We are—for the most part—a risk-averse management group, perhaps one of the most conservative within American enterprise. Second, although the strategies may not be completely new, they are not widely practiced. In some cases, they are not even minimally practiced in this industry. Yet, as I mention throughout the book, they *are* widely practiced and highly regarded in other industries nation- and worldwide.

That pervasive practice is the perspective I bring to this forum and is one of my main reasons for writing this book. My career began outside of healthcare. I started in the consumer goods industry with a well-respected subsidiary of a Fortune 100 firm. When I migrated to healthcare in the mid-1980s, I was struck most by how little we borrow from other industries and how much we have to gain by doing so. Fundamentally, this book is all about that basic precept—looking without to improve within.

As this book is being written, major organizations and credible individuals are calling for fundamental restructuring of the healthcare system. As markets expand, technologies advance, and the world shrinks, many ask why healthcare has not yet transitioned to the third millennium. The best designers and architects for the changes needed are those who know the industry from the inside but who are willing to expand their view, enlarge their horizon, and broaden their perspective. In essence, those who need to revamp and reform are not the rookies, the pundits, or the politicians, but the in-house experts.

My goal in presenting these strategies is not necessarily to single-handedly nor expeditiously turn the supertanker we call healthcare around and get it back on course. Rather, this book is written for forward-thinking, risk-taking, even "adventure"-loving executives who want to put a little excitement into their daily routine and maybe add some margin to their bottom line. In the process, one or two organizations may just come up with a new approach for a breakthrough delivery model that helps fulfill their mission, strengthen the overall system, and preserve the free-market structure. Stranger things have happened.

Introduction

*You don't have to be rich and famous to be
happy. Rich is enough.*

—Alan Alda

BACKGROUND

Healthcare is on a high wire. The industry is faced with daunting challenges presented by declining reimbursement, increasing federal intervention, and diminishing public support and
perception. At the same time, many hospitals are in such ten-
uous financial straits that they have neither the resources nor
the energy to thoroughly analyze these issues and successfully
resolve them. It is not the best of times for health systems and
hospitals, and the future does not look very promising.

Many organizations will have difficulty resolving their problems before they succumb to closure, bankruptcy, or consolidation. If healthcare remains private over the next decade—a
prospect that some seriously question—the number of providers
that remain could diminish by as much as one-fifth. Many of
those that do remain solvent will do so based on their deep
cash reserves and their ability to draw on financial resources

outside of traditional operating income streams. And some—a select group—will recognize the turbulent waters, navigate them successfully, and actually come out of the present market storms better off than before. These organizations will have leadership that is proactive, aggressive, and innovative. This book is written for those organizations and the individuals who lead them.

LOCAL SOLUTIONS FOR LOCALLY MANAGED ORGANIZATIONS

This book is not about global solutions, industrywide opportunities, or broad-reaching efforts to save American healthcare. Rather, the book is about taking reasonable risks and pursuing innovative strategies. Some healthcare professionals have difficulty accepting and embracing innovative thinking or adopting strategies that have not been proven over the years and throughout the industry. Healthcare is sometimes referred to as a "me-too" or lemming industry; organizations tend to jump on the strategy bandwagon. Examples of this may be witnessed in the major push in the mid- to late 1990s to achieve vertical integration with physicians. Now, in retrospect, that strategy seems to be fundamentally flawed, as many organizations have witnessed serious financial losses and precipitous declines in operating income as a result of the ill-fated strategy.

Many Americans are not aware of the serious managerial and economic challenges this industry currently experiences. In truth, most of our fellow citizens have little understanding of how the industry works. In fact, even some people in healthcare do not have a firm grip on it. The healthcare system is complex, change resistant, and hierarchical. Thus, when healthcare professionals and industry advocates try to make a case for government assistance, employer understanding, or public support, the pleas often fall on deaf or disinterested ears.

Industry survivors will recognize that their fate is in their own hands and will not rely on industry associations, government representatives, or market serendipity. Those organizations that look to others for resolution will soon find that they are in the same position as the two vagabonds in Samuel Beckett's classic play, *Waiting for Godot*. Throughout the entire play, the two protagonists await the mysterious and elusive Godot, who never does arrive. So it will likely be for some healthcare organizations. For too many organizations and individuals, the cavalry is not coming to the rescue; to paraphrase the classic line from the comic strip *Pogo*, "We have met the cavalry and it is us."

Thus, I designed this book to assist the in-residence cavalry and to give forward-thinking, risk-taking healthcare executives a few ideas for boosting the bottom line and preserving their organization's financial health. Again, whereas many of these ideas may be well known, few are widely practiced. As author Stephen Covey is known to say when critics argue that his concepts (from his best-selling book *The 7 Habits of Highly Effective People*) are merely common sense, "Maybe so, but common sense is not common practice."

DRAWING ON OTHER INDUSTRY EXPERIENCE

These strategies are definitely not common practice, nor will they become so any time soon. They call for viewing healthcare from a different angle and approaching its operations with a varied perspective. However, this perspective is not unique in American enterprise. Many of the concepts outlined in this book parallel the practices of other U. S. industries. In fact, in some respects, healthcare is the outsider when it comes to business practices. Those who argue that healthcare is market driven have probably not spent much time in or attention to other market-driven industries in the current global economy. Recent articles in the trade press have called attention to this disconcerting practice of delaying acceptance of otherwise common business practices. In fact, some have postulated that advanced information technology may in fact be the catalyst to bring healthcare up to speed and in sync with other American enterprise.

I take that premise one step further and argue that all of these strategies can be good catalysts for enhancing an organization's bottom line by improving its operational performance. These strategies can also be the means by which we as professional managers take greater control of our financial destiny. These principles or strategies have, for the most part, been tested and proven in other industries and in pioneering organizations within our own industry. Consequently, this is not theory but proven practice and sound strategy.

Thus, some may find this book slightly different from other healthcare management books on strategy. Admittedly, it may require a somewhat different mind-set and an innovative array of skill sets. Yet stepping outside our traditional and comfortable boundaries and exploring reasonable strategies that can propel our organizations into the future and help maintain their financial stability is a good thing. Nonetheless, market-based approaches and practices are sometimes difficult to understand and even more challenging to execute for some healthcare executives.

As proof of this theory, I offer my experience in the late 1980s. I coauthored a book on product line management with a colleague and friend, Jim Folger. The book was published by the American Hospital Association and, by industry standards, was quite well received. However, the premise of the book was that product line management (now termed service line management within the industry) was an organizational imperative, not a marketing initiative. Despite our best efforts, we were not able to successfully persuade many people that the concept should be applied organizationwide, not specific to function. Consequently, many who read the book missed its main focus, and product line management became a marketing fad that fizzled.

This is entirely understandable. Many senior executives were schooled on and grounded in a field where the medical model (also deemed "expert model") ruled. In that model, experts diagnose, then prescribe. Reimbursement was not regulated by market forces but rather flowed from cost-plus sources or third-party payers.

BECOMING A MARKET-DRIVEN INDUSTRY

A true market-driven environment is altogether different. No automatic reimbursement mechanism exists. Rather, the acquisition of the product is driven by the demands of the customer and the value the customer places on the product or service. In healthcare, determining the customer is somewhat problematic. Over time, the economic clout or influence of those customers has shifted. For example, one could argue that the two most important customer groups in the healthcare industry are the government and major employers. (In consumer-oriented industries, the consumer is the individual or entity that is also the end user or one who "consumes" the product; the customer is the one who purchases the product.)

Ask most healthcare executives who the "customer" is, and they will respond with "physicians," "managed care organizations," or "patients." This limited prioritization is further validated by the amount of time healthcare professionals spend with these groups, as opposed to employer representatives or government operatives. If you ask healthcare executives how much time they spend discussing strategy or spending time with employers or government agencies that administer payment, they will likely give you blank stares. Much of the strategy outlined within the ensuing pages therefore deals with employers, government agencies, and policymakers.

This premise was proven in a meeting with individuals who represented the largest employers in Texas. They were meeting to form a healthcare business coalition in Austin. During the course of the meeting, I realized they did not trust healthcare leaders and did not want them at the table as they formed the coalition. Now, one could reasonably ask, "What other industry in America would find customers unwilling to have its manufacturers at the table as they discuss the industry's paradigm for the future?" Yet that was exactly the stance of this group, and it indicated where we are as leaders—trying to stave off powerful individuals and organizations that would push us toward centralized healthcare and federalized medicine. Many business executives who represent millions of covered lives have simply lost faith in the current operating system as it relates to healthcare delivery. Furthermore, they are not about to invite healthcare leaders to the table to discuss solutions—only to implement mandates once they develop them.

OVERVIEW OF THE BOOK

Another major difference between market-driven industries and healthcare is the immutability of products and services. In most industries in the United States—technology, financial services, retail products—extensive turnover and replacement of the goods and services offered takes place. That is not the case in healthcare. This industry has what I call the medical superglue effect, which is the incredible "stickiness" for services even if they do not produce favorable bottom lines. In fact, this book begins with the call to consolidate and streamline. That one principle is fundamental—as other industries have already learned—because you cannot "make it up on volume"; organizations cannot effectively expand if they continue to offer the same number of services with the same number of people to oversee them.

The only organization that can effectively grow and expand is one that is committed to a consistent evaluation of its service lines and the routine divestiture, consolidation, or abandonment of poor performers. If a healthcare facility can never get to the point of thinning down, it can never effectively bulk up. The organization that is consistently and continuously evaluating its operating portfolio is the one most likely to be aligned with market trends and customer needs. That is a hallmark of successful organizations in every other industry and should become a standard operating practice for all organizations that want to remain viable and provide highly valued services.

I also devote considerable time and attention to two relatively new strategies for healthcare, effectively using the Internet as a management tool and marshalling the concept of "co-opetition." Co-opetition—a combination of competition and cooperation—is not actually a new concept in American industry, especially for the field of technology, but for the healthcare industry it is significantly innovative. Utilizing both notions of the Internet and co-opetition offers the best hope for this industry and may prove to be the elements of enterprise that preserve the free-market model for this nation.

Finally, some chapters are devoted to opportunities that may seem marginal in their promise of additional income: broadening the market by providing reasonable and practical access for the uninsured, expanding the management portfolio to the entire field of complementary medicine, and building an enterprise of retail and visual traffic. Some may maintain that these strategies are nominally effective in producing significant incremental revenue. However, these strategies represent a discipline and a process that is necessary and invaluable. Although they may not produce the kind of immediate results and revenue streams that expansion of cardiology or obstetric services do, they offer the forceful dynamic that results from modifying the organization's portfolio of services, pursuing a different operational angle, and learning to operate in a new milieu.

NEW MIND-SET FOR THE THIRD MILLENNIUM

Therein lies the rationale for, as well as the genius in, such exploration. That many healthcare organizations will fail in their execution of complementary medicine, for example, is given. The idea is not without merit, but the execution is flawed and uninspiring. The organizations that will immediately survive and ultimately thrive are those that know how to pursue these unconventional strategies by bringing in individuals with different approaches, exploring and executing innovative strategies, and providing those services that the market demands and customers desire.

Fundamentally, this is a book about change that is both healthy and essential. We participate in an economy that demands constant and rapid change. To remain viable, the industry and its individual organizations must prove capable of embracing the concept of change and implementing the kind of worthwhile and productive adjustments that improve operations. Ultimately, that may prove the difference between those readers who will find this book merely interesting and those who will find it invigorating, productive, and profitable. Here's to the latter.

1

Streamline Operations Through Service Line Management[1]

Truth is, most of us are spread too thin.

—Bertrand Russell

HEALTHCARE ORGANIZATIONS HAVE become known for providing the widest array of services possible. Perhaps the time has come to abandon that traditional model and scale back to become more efficient and economically viable. Looking forward, one of the biggest challenges healthcare executives will face is committing to and handling the elimination of marginally producing service lines. The key is to trim down prior to a directive from consultants in response to a financial crisis, an eleventh-hour mandate from the board of directors, or a coerced downsizing prompted by a temporary turnaround firm. This type of rapid-fire downsizing, either in terms of personnel or product lines, is overly reactive and usually suboptimal.

Why is the successful application of service line management such a rarity in our ranks? Is it likely to remain so over the next several years? As some management experts have noted, reviewing the barriers to progress prior to describing the pathways to success is sometimes helpful. Aware of such hurdles—historic and perhaps even endemic—informed leaders might be more likely to correct their course and implement the necessary initiatives required to propel their organizations into the future.

BIGGER IS NOT NECESSARILY BETTER

First, some healthcare executives are under the mistaken notion that bigger is better. The overused and now tritely glib phrase "edifice complex" is perhaps more indigenous to the healthcare industry than any other enterprise sector in the United States. Indeed, building expansion and medical campus extension appear to be part of the healthcare DNA. This seeming predisposition (call it the "architectural chromosome") toward expansion is understandable given the economic history of healthcare, which (because of cost-plus reimbursement) encouraged and rewarded increased organizational overhead. What better way to increase overhead than to expand physical capacity and offer more services?

However, that financial payment structure and subsequent stream of cash flow have been all but extinct for nearly two decades. Healthcare is a supertanker that takes a long time and a great deal of effort to turn, but twenty years is a long time to take to change course. Nonetheless, as one tries to determine why healthcare executives continue to expand physical facilities in an information-age economy, we are forced to trace the answer back to the origin of the industry.

The investigative reporters who exposed the Watergate wiretapping scandal, Bob Woodward and Carl Bernstein, were told to "follow the money." For many of the current senior executives in healthcare, the path to more money has historically been increased physical capacity. It therefore seems to be a mind-set that is deeply engrained and thus not easily displaced.

Someone inspecting this industry from outside its cultural confines might be baffled as to why seemingly bright healthcare executives continue to remain so fixated on expanding services when it appears to makes little sense and demands such heavy monetary investment. This could be called mental model inertia and will likely prove the bane of individuals and organizations that fail to adapt to new economies and complex environments. This fixation on growth for growth's sake must be modified. Over the past five to ten years far too many healthcare executives have incurred serious debt and endangered their organization's ability to survive by continuing in that outdated approach.

Admittedly, some of this most recent fervor for expansion was precipitated by the out-of-control growth of for-profit chains modeled after Wal-Mart. During the early years of the 1990s, the larger investor-owned chains pursued a growth strategy that was unprecedented and ultimately unsustainable. In response, merger and acquisition activity skyrocketed in both the for-profit and not-for-profit sectors. The extreme example of this on the not-for-profit side was the Allegheny Health, Education and Research Foundation (AHERF) in Pennsylvania. AHERF was the poster child for not-for-profit expansion and thus the great counterbalance to the Columbia/HCA and Tenet organizations. That was the case, at least, until the operational wheels came off for AHERF and the large system was forced to face financial reality and file for Chapter 11 bankruptcy.

The AHERF debacle taught the industry many lessons, but perhaps the most important was that neither saving grace nor economic stability results from ill-conceived and uncontrolled growth. AHERF precipitously fell from high-profile prototype to the position of unwitting and unwanted example of rapid self-destruction. Although AHERF may be somewhat isolated in its rapid-rise-to-dramatic-fall cycle (further punctuated by lawsuits, criminal indictments, and required financial bailout), many other systems caught expansion fever and have suffered, or will suffer, the painful side effects of the "growth is great" illusion.

Second, some healthcare executives have a sense that if they do not provide the service, their competition might have an advantage over them. The prevailing sentiment is that patients and physicians will opt for the organization that provides the broadest array of services. Such logic is fundamentally flawed.

For most services, doctors still select the hospital or healthcare provider. Consequently, the notion of "one-stop shopping" does not hold the promise that its promoters gave it. For the most part, doctors are specialty specific. They do not refer their patients to Hospital X or Health System Y because they have every service under the sun. They refer or admit their patients to a particular hospital because it has the most advanced equipment, the best nurses, the most qualified medical staff, or — and this is the key reason — the most convenient location. This long-held logic was proven by extensive research conducted by the Healthcare Advisory Board in 1998. Conducting rather sophisticated market research, known as conjoint analysis, the Advisory Board produced survey results that clearly proved geographic convenience, or proximity to a facility, is far and away the number one reason doctors select hospitals (Healthcare Advisory Board 1999).

Along that line, many industry insiders became irritated a few years ago when some high-profile healthcare executives said they wanted to be the Wal-Mart of healthcare. Such disdain was appropriate. Healthcare is not much like retailing, so comparisons to Wal-Mart, Sears, or Dillards are a stretch, if not far-fetched. So too is the concept of one-stop shopping with its cry for expanded service lines and extensive product or service offerings.

Furthermore, health plans give very little, if any, quarter or leverage to systems that have all the services in the galaxy. This lack of negotiating clout as a result of comprehensiveness has been exposed and defrocked through countless cases involving niche players or smaller hospitals. The concept of scale equating to increased leverage at the negotiating table may be a fascinating theory, but it has not proven verifiable.

The third reason healthcare executives are ineffective in dropping or consolidating entire service lines is the lack of reliable data. Even in this age when a global positioning system can pinpoint an individual's location (within inches) anywhere on earth, most healthcare executives cannot say if their cardiology department makes a higher margin than their orthopedics service line. This dearth of reliable data and shameful lack of good cost accounting programs have been the bane of decision makers in this industry for three decades. Although some pioneers have made impressive progress, too many executives appear to be mired in mediocre information technology (IT) systems that produce spurious or inconclusive data.

THE STREAMLINE IMPERATIVE

Why should a health system go against its generic grain and begin consolidating or liquidating service lines? The answer is easy: *to survive.* Organizations that fail to constrict or consolidate will falter and fail. It is that simple. Organizational growth patterns are like pruning trees. The most successful gardeners know that healthy trees and bushes require periodic pruning — scaling the tree or bush back to allow new growth so that it becomes more robust. The difference between the pruning analogy and healthcare organizations is that pruning is not as selective. Healthcare leaders must eliminate certain sections of their organization so they can focus their efforts on the sections that matter most and produce the highest economic returns and social benefits. Unfortunately, many executives never get to the pruning stage and consequently are likely to sacrifice the entire organization by maintaining a large, overwhelmingly inefficient, and outdated system.

Healthcare executives who are incapable of streamlining their organization are unwilling to let go. By holding onto everything within their grasp, they may endanger their organization financially and strategically. Their Achilles' heel is likely the marginally efficient service line, the internally developed program, or perhaps a particular pet project—any or all of which may have long since lost their value to the organization.

The very process of streamlining is essential to successful development of new business opportunities and future service line expansion. One can observe rather quickly in this field that too many executives pursue new opportunities with the same old cadre of managers. This "piling on" of responsibilities often results in an organization with burned-out managers and misappropriated resources. More often than not, the new business consumes time, energy, and focus—and it usually produces fewer favorable results than the existing business. The new venture is labeled a nonperformer and the manager in charge is tainted with failure.

By streamlining, the organization is capable of pursuing new opportunities with the appropriate individuals ("fresh blood") and adequate resources. Most things done on a shoe-string budget are neither worth the effort nor the exercise. They look cheap, they start wrong, and they damage the individuals associated with such projects. Taking a few million dollars out of the organization, committing some of that money to new ventures, and giving the carefully planned initiatives every chance of success is a far better solution. If an organization is not willing to exercise that kind of discipline, it should not attempt to develop new opportunities or expand into new markets.

SEVEN STEPS TO STREAMLINING

1. Embrace the Attitude that Svelte Is Better

Many healthcare managers and executives have difficulty coming to terms with the notion that a leaner organization is often a healthier one. Healthcare enterprises have come to view organizational girth as a benefit when the opposite is true. Far too many leaders assess their institution's value on a breadth scale, rather than on a financial depth scale. Thus, shifting out of the former attitude to one of considering the possibility of systematically slimming down will not be an easy task, but it is the necessary first step.

One good motivator that may facilitate this change of mindset is the relatively recent surge in niche players, or specialty-specific healthcare organizations, that concentrate on one or two service lines. These specialized organizations usually focus on highly profitable service lines such as cardiology, obstetrics, or orthopedics. They are able to carve out these lines both in terms of isolating the scope of their services and positioning their organization uppermost in the minds of the consumers. They have taken a chapter from retail specialty stores and applied it successfully to healthcare. In one Southwest city, an upstart specialty hospital focusing on cardiology was able to rapidly vault ahead of its two much larger and better established health systems and lodge its position firmly in the minds of consumers. In this particular market, researchers asked respondents to name a hospital or health system that excelled in a particular service line. For all categories except cardiology, the differentiation was basically nonexistent, with the most common response being "I don't know." For cardiology services, however, this specialty hospital was able to claim a commanding 50 percent preference after only two years in the market.

This example illustrates that organizations that believe indistinguishable breadth will carry the day in a skirmish with a skillful specialty player will probably be proven wrong. And although the financial viability of specialty players has not yet been determined, their rapid rise and impressive inroads into many markets should serve as a wake-up call to large systems that mere girth is not enough to win the battle for individual service lines.

At the same time, unprofitable lines are a financial drain and a management distraction. Given all the challenges and pressing issues that healthcare leaders face in these turbulent times, we cannot afford the luxury of accommodating service lines that do not pull their economic weight and that drag down the rest of the organization, exhausting its management team and weakening its overall strength. Consequently, the first step on the liberating road to streamlining is recognizing that svelte is better if the trimming down can be done in a systematic and semiscientific manner.

2. Develop the Criteria for Evaluating Service Lines

How does a decision maker determine which lines to trim back or discard? Most important is establishing objective criteria by which the organization can evaluate its service lines. This is not necessarily an easy task, and many organizations falter when they try to establish standardized criteria, but it has been done successfully and impressively. Granted, some organizations have more inherent capabilities in this regard due to more extensive and accurate cost accounting systems, but nearly all organizations can develop criteria, even if they are not as refined and calculated as others.

In evaluating the efficacy of service lines, the patently obvious first step is to identify the service lines themselves. Despite the seeming sensibility of this, the process breaks down at this stage for many healthcare organizations because few in the organization will agree at the outset what criteria will be used. The simple issue of "just how does the enterprise determine its service lines" is not simple at all.

Various factions within an organization will often promote definitions that are obscure, random, and indiscriminate. For example, in the heat of the criteria establishment session, someone will argue that pastoral care should be a service line. Not wanting to offend anyone, the group may agree. Then an ardent advocate of volunteer services will assert a claim for that area, and before long, the hospital has identified 45 service lines, most of which have nothing in common to measure and no standard set of accountability criteria on which to assess the viability of each line. This scenario has repeated itself countless times across the nation for over two decades now.

Yet its proliferation does not justify its application. This kind of broad-range approach to service line management does the organization little good and will usually result in more frustration than benefit. When no (or few) common evaluative criteria exist, there is little accountability and consequently no objective way to eliminate or expand particular service lines based on true merit and overall benefit to the organization. Therefore, I recommend that the organization determine at the outset that service lines will be limited to disease categories (at least to get started) and that the entire universe be limited to no more than seven to ten lines. The rest go into a reserve pool to be evaluated later. Will that ruffle some feathers? Will that cause some department managers to feel underappreciated? Will such internal conflict offset the gains from the streamlining exercise? Yes, yes, and I seriously doubt it.

However, if an organization's management team believes that a serious effort of streamlining via service line management will have everyone's consensus, the process is best not started at all. We are, after all, talking about systematic and methodical reduction—of services, of departments, and of people. Although the systematic determination of service lines may seem a bit mercenary, it is actually far better than a random, reactionary, and counterproductive reduction of force in the form of across-the-board layoffs or expedient elimination of services. The latter is the norm, but it is not a healthy norm.

Although a few good criteria for measuring service lines exist, the oldest and arguably most universal is diagnosis-related group (DRG) classification. Shortly after DRGs were established in the mid-1980s, accounting firms developed the means to identify and isolate service lines. Using DRGs as a classification system is helpful because the data are, for the most part, available from a number of sources. Furthermore, since the data are reported in a standard format, national data companies can assess the effectiveness of one hospital's service line against its competitors in the same market. National benchmarks can also factor into the evaluation equation, measured against best practices of the leading hospitals and health systems.

DRG classification has limitations. It focuses on inpatient volume and therefore neglects or underestimates outpatient measures. Also, separating out more complex service lines such as oncology is difficult. Furthermore, hospitals—nationally as well as in local markets—report their data with little third-party verification; hence, the data are only as valid as the individual who reports them to the clearinghouse organization or regulatory body.

That said, DRGs are still a good basic and relatively universal system of assessment and measurement. The danger in arguing the faults of DRG classification is that it misrepresents the probable alternatives, becoming a straw man argument with no reasonable substitute. In essence, those who argue that DRGs are not accurate enough, too arcane, or inconclusive unwittingly may defeat the entire initiative by lobbying for an idyllic but nonexistent substitute. This is another scenario that has played itself out many times throughout the country. For example, an organization may get hopelessly hung up on how to define the oncology service line and in their interminable delay forestall the service line initiative into an early demise.

A far better approach for most organizations is to begin with a DRG evaluation. As the organization progresses and becomes more adept at the basic concept of service line management, it can incorporate more accurate or refined data. The key is to identify the service lines and begin the process. Fine tuning can occur well into the initiative.

3. Assign Service Line Managers to Each Line

Once the seven to ten service lines have been established, the next step is to assign a manager or director to each line. This does not need to be a soul-searching, heart-rending process. There was a time—back in the late 1980s—when some service line gurus, consultants, or both (they are not necessarily the same thing) recommended hiring managers from outside the ranks. Given the Spartan times in the industry now and the need for rapid-fire implementation, the optimal, if not fundamentally easier, strategy is to hire people from inside the organization who are qualified by nature of their familiarity with it. The cardiology service line manager could be the director of nursing for that area, the head of the catheterization laboratory, or a vice president who has responsibility for cardiac services. The person should be someone familiar with the people, the equipment, and the operation of that line. In part, the rationale of some experts for hiring outside service line managers was to give the line a fresh perspective, a new look, a consumer's viewpoint. However, that applied more to the marketing effort, and given that service line management is more operationally based than marketing oriented, assigning someone familiar with the operational nuances of the area is a better solution.

These managers should understand that, although they may still have other duties to perform within the organization, they will be assessed (and I recommend) compensated based on achieving the objectives of their service line. The latter is an important clarification, as bottom-line performance may not be the only measure that counts. For example, if in the audit stage of service line assessment (discussed in step 4, below) the organization decides downsizing, merging, or jettisoning a particular line is in its best interest, the service line manager should be rewarded for successfully completing that objective. This is a very important differentiation, the misunderstanding of which often hinders the overall process.

Too many organizations that embark on the service line path gauge success only by traditional measures—increased volume, improved profitability, and greater market share. However, that assumes all service lines are like the children in Lake Wobegon—above average—and therefore each line merits expansion. Such a belief is not only a fallacy, it undermines the service line effort, as such an attitude never produces the previously mentioned concentration on the true stellar performers nor the diminishment or abandonment of those lines that are past their prime.

Hence, this provides another good reason for hiring service line mangers from within and converting their jobs. Someone coming from outside the organization will not be excited about eliminating the service or department that he or she oversees. However, a vice president who has responsibility for several lines or departments will not be as remiss to reduce or eliminate one particular line, especially if the organization has identified that objective early in the process.

In addition to assigning service line managers, the organization should also form multidisciplinary teams for each area. This serves several purposes, not the least of which is involving more people within the hospital or health system in the overall process. Additionally, a multidisciplinary team, functioning under a matrix structure, will provide broader perspective and enhance the decision-making process as strategy is developed. Finally, a team structure will facilitate implementation of tactics identified in the plan, as a crossfunctional team assures greater buy-in and cooperation throughout the organization.

The team should meet as frequently as necessary—monthly is usually sufficient—with the service line manager serving as the head of the team. The team should include clinical staff or managers from that particular discipline, as well as support staff, such as finance, marketing, and administration. Ancillary staff, such as those from laboratories or radiology departments, should also be considered. However, the team should be kept at a reasonable size, with no more than seven to ten members. Otherwise, people will feel they are merely passively participating and not making a contribution. Teams that try to include too broad a spectrum usually run the risk of having two or three strong-willed people dominate the meetings and control the direction. That is more difficult to do when only seven or eight members are on the team and everyone is expected to be a contributor.

4. Conduct a Service Line Audit and Array the Lines by Evaluative Criteria

Once the evaluative criteria are determined, the service lines are selected, and the managers are assigned, the next step is to conduct an audit. This is done after the managers are selected because they may need to get involved in gathering and validating the data. This process serves two purposes. First and foremost, it helps familiarize the individual manager with his or her service line based on the criteria selected for evaluation. Second, it spreads the load in terms of gathering and verifying the data. Fortunately, many department heads, nursing managers, and administrative officers are already familiar with some of this data.

The systematic gathering, validating, and publishing of the data will be beneficial in and of itself. Simply initiating the process will be both illuminating and liberating—not to mention beneficial to the bottom line. This has been the experience for several healthcare executives who, after completing this process either in a rather rudimentary way or in sophisticated fashion have wondered why they did not start sooner.

Given that many hospitals or health systems are still lagging in their ability to get good cost accounting data, the first approach assumes that the organization cannot separate the financial winners from the economic deadwood. At the least, they are not able to do so on contribution margin or some measure of financial viability that is understood and applied in every business school in the United States. It is not the only factor, but a financial assessment is at the heart of first-phase analysis. Financial evaluation is key when arraying service lines in, for example, a portfolio grid. Another good measure for evaluating the lines that can serve as the other axis on the portfolio grid could be relative volume. Both these measures should be relatively easy to obtain, especially if the organization is using a measure as standard as DRGs. Another possible measure, which is admittedly slightly more subjective, is growth potential. This can be assessed based on such quantitative measures as three-year trend lines, as well as subjective measures such as competitive entrances and exits, medical staff considerations, marketing campaigns, or any other more qualitative factors.

Once the data have been gathered for each service line, all the lines can be depicted in a graphic format that visually displays the relative strengths, weaknesses, and opportunities for the organization's core services. Using the three criteria mentioned above, an organization could develop a portfolio analysis or grid similar to the one shown in Figure 1.1. This grid

FIGURE 1.1: SERVICE LINE PORTFOLIO GRID—
CONTRIBUTION AND EASE OF CONSOLIDATION/
ELIMINATION

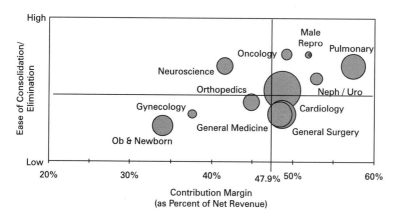

depicts the financial strength of each line on the *x*-axis, with the lines with the highest contribution margin positioned on the far right. The *y*-axis is a more subjective measure of the potential for consolidating or eliminating the line, with the upper areas of the grid representing greater ease in restructuring. In this example, obstetrics would be the line most difficult to eliminate or consolidate, while oncology represents the line with the greatest likelihood for diminishment or restructuring.

The size of each service line is a measure of its relative revenue position; hence, in this example, cardiology is the largest service line, as well as being one of the more profitable lines. These kinds of grids are also called bubble charts or two-axis matrices and derive from the famous "growth-share matrix" popularized by the Boston Consulting Group in the 1960s. They establish an organization average (in this case 47.9 percent for contribution margin to fixed costs) and depict how each individual service line stacks up against the organization average.

These grids can have any number of variables on the axes. Typically, they show a financial measure (e.g., revenue, contribution margin, or profit) and an external competitive measure (e.g., market share, growth potential, or consolidation/elimination probability).

Once the audit or evaluation is conducted and the service lines are arrayed in this format, or some similar configuration, the executive can assess strategy going forward for each service line. The value of such a graphical representation is twofold. First, one can see in a moment where the organization is both strong and potentially vulnerable. In the example shown in Figure 1.1, this organization is highly dependent on just a few service lines for its profitability. Should competitive forces, changes in government reimbursement, or managed care pricing pressures hit one or two of these lines hard, the organization will have a tough time recovering. The strategy for these service lines, then, is to protect where needed and expand where possible.

At the same time, this organization has a fair number of marginal performers. These lines could be evaluated for improvement in the financial performance of the line. Is the weak performance a function of volume? Do they carry unnecessary costs? Could a possible consolidation with another market player make a particular line more economically viable?

The second reason for graphically displaying the identified service lines in such a way is that it establishes a baseline for future evaluation and comparison. Visualizing progress or digression is far easier using this method when assessing multiple lines. This point recalls the original premise that hospitals and health systems need to subdivide their organizations into strategic business units. By so doing, they are more apt to meet the demands of the market and counteract the encroachment of competitors, especially niche players. A portfolio grid provides a clear visual picture of the organization as it exists, as well as how it has changed over time.

5. Determine Strategy as an Organization

Once the audit is completed, the lines arrayed, and the graphic displayed, the next step is to determine strategy organizationally, not independently. This step is often overlooked or neglected as the individual service line managers battle to emerge as king of the hill and victor of the most market share. However, such unorganized, ill-coordinated, and random pursuit of individual service line success is suboptimal. This is one important area where healthcare differs from some manufacturing and retailing concerns. Many of those enterprises adopt, perhaps appropriately, a mentality supporting every line for itself. That may work well for a company such as Procter & Gamble or General Electric, but healthcare has too much interconnectedness—just like the human body—for such an uncoordinated approach.

A clear understanding is necessary at the outset as to what criteria matter the most and what is most relevant for the organization going forward. Only then can the organization achieve its overall strategic goals by ensuring that the individual lines are pursuing objectives that align with and support the overall direction. And such goals must be more than merely financial. Otherwise, the means to get to the end may damage the enterprise. Thus, the portfolio grid is only one tool for assessment and strategy. It is largely based on economic performance and growth potential. However, each organization must decide what other criteria factor into the evaluation of a successful service line for it.

One example of this is women's services, specifically obstetrics. Consider two actual case studies of the misapplication of this principle: The first was a for-profit chain in the early 1980s that conducted a thorough financial analysis of service line profitability and determined that OB/GYN was near the bottom in terms of reimbursement. Consequently, this chain opened a hospital in southern Washington state without birthing services. Little time passed before the executives in charge of the facility (and the chain) realized that a new hospital in a modest-sized market would not be very successful without offering women's services. They scrambled to retrofit the hospital and add OB services but lost critical time, early success, and community perception as a full-service hospital.

The other example comes from another for-profit hospital. This facility was designed to be a specialty hospital — in this case, orthopedics. It was a moderately sized facility and the third hospital in a three-hospital city, drawing over three-fourths of its volume from outside the immediate confines of the community. During its first few years, it performed well, receiving an adequate number of patients with high-margin surgeries and aligned services. However, as managed care came to that market and intermediaries began negotiating "package deals" with companies, this particular hospital found itself carved out of more contracts because it did not offer a broad array of services to companies to make it attractive. Again, in an effort to adjust to market pressures and consumer demands, the organization attempted to restructure, by retooling and renovating, to offer OB services. In this case, however, the late entry into the critical line of women's services, coupled with fiercely intense market pressures, made recovering the lost ground nearly impossible for the hospitals. Ultimately, it was consolidated into one of the other two health systems in the area.

The point in these two situations is that every organization should be careful to not focus solely on economics. Borrowing a term from retailing, some service lines are "loss leaders." These are essential to every business in every industry. Organizations that abandon their core services, or their loss leaders, because they do not produce the economic returns, rue the day they pursued such a shortsighted strategy.

Therefore, in all the analysis, a clear realization is necessary *up front* that financial evaluation is a possible starting point, but that evaluation is not the only criteria by which service lines (or departments or whatever unit of measure is adopted) are reviewed. This may seem overly simplistic; however, if it is not well understood at the outset, the willingness to provide data as well as the objectivity with which it is evaluated will be gravely hindered. If department managers firmly believe the only criteria that matters in their survival is economic performance, an effort—conscious or not—to either distort the data or challenge its reliability will be felt. The resulting theatrics and gymnastics will consume valuable time and deplete organizational resources.

The main benefit of an organizationwide strategy will be to more carefully monitor activity so that duplication is avoided, superfluous activity is reduced, and resources are maximized. The service lines are like individual battalions, but the bigger battle must be envisioned at a higher level. Otherwise, some of the lower potential service lines may consume a disproportionate share of management time and organizational resources. This happens often in hospitals and health systems that fail to coordinate strategy at the higher level and ensure (or at least encourage) aligned goals at the department and service line level.

A basic evaluation of financial strength by product line begins with two data points—a top line net revenue and a bottom line calculation. For the latter, the hospital could use operating income, net income, or earnings before interest, taxes, and depreciation and amortization (EBITDA). The bottom line calculation will likely depend on which number the organization typically reports to the board of directors and will largely be determined by the organization's status. For-profit concerns, for example, base most of their financial calculations on EBITDA (or EBDITA, depending on which accounting firm they use and which acronym the company likes the best).

Service line consultants recommend a trend analysis of at least three years for such an evaluation. Data from one year clearly do not reflect the market status and may result in abnormal results and suboptimal decision making. If available, a five-year analysis is preferable and will provide a thorough look at the organization's trended performance for its service line as well as give some enlightening data for expected future performance.

The service line revenue and profitability calculations can then be arrayed in a number of venues, ranging from a simple bar chart arrangement to a more sophisticated dual-axis portfolio grid as depicted earlier in this chapter. This becomes the baseline tool for beginning the discussion, and based on the experience of others, it will likely be a lively discussion.

Some might reasonably ask, "But what if your organization doesn't even have the capacity to determine how to divide up its service lines?" Even now many organizations still do not have that capacity. Several options are available to such organizations.

One option is to obtain a standard DRG definition of service lines (at least for the acute care component) and use that as a basis. Such a definition can be obtained from most of the Big Five accounting firms. Arthur Andersen did pioneering work in this field in the 1980s; most firms have adopted a definition that is more easily applicable. Several companies and independent consultants also specialize in developing service line definitions and classifications, and some nationally known data companies focus on establishing and measuring service lines. These names can be gleaned from a consulting reference guide or by asking peers within the industry who have pursued this path previously. Numerous conferences on the subject of service line management are available, as it has experienced a revival in the past few years. These conferences often showcase organizations and individuals that specialize in the field of service line management. Books on the subject as well as numerous articles are also available.[2]

Once the data are obtained, the numbers should be arrayed in a spreadsheet format, from top to bottom and divided into quadrants, with the bottom two quadrants (in terms of income performance) highlighted as the starting point for consideration. This becomes the launching pad for developing strategies for dealing with these underperforming service lines or assessing their nonfinancial value in the overall portfolio.

If an organization does not have ready access to such numbers in house, it can conduct a more thorough analysis that encompasses other quantitative factors (more than revenues and bottom-line calculations). These would include components such as growth trends, market share potential, and complement value to other service lines. These numerical considerations could be diagramed in a multidimensional graph or grid such as the bubble chart displayed in Figure 1.1. This provides a visual illustration of the relative position of each of the service lines in the context of more variables than just top-line and bottom-line financial performance. It also provides a sense of dynamic perspective over a few years rather than a stagnant snapshot in time. One big mistake that many healthcare executives make in evaluating service line performance is to review recent history or present performance rather than couch the analysis in terms of future potential. In doing this, executives may commit the egregious (but not uncommon) error of discarding or downsizing tomorrow's brightest opportunity for today's budgetary mandate. A more sophisticated analysis with other key benchmarks, such as growth potential or market share trends, tends to diffuse the natural (but dangerous) tendency to regard and review services in a vacuum or a narrowly defined viewpoint.

Another way to incorporate multiple variables into the analysis is to assign a numerical weight to each variable. Although this is admittedly subjective, it serves to encompass more factors than just the two financial components. For example, in evaluating service lines, the equation could include the five variables as listed below:

A = net revenue;
B = operating income;
C = market share (current);
D = growth potential in percent (over five years); and
E = economic contribution to other lines.

Each one of these variables is assigned a weight. For simplicity's sake, I give each one a weight of 20 percent, or 0.2. All the service lines are arrayed in performance quadrants for each variable. For example, if an organization is evaluating eight service lines, the top two performers in net revenue are in the top quadrant and assigned a value of 4 for that variable. The two next best performing service lines would be in the next quadrant and assigned a value of 3 for net revenue.

The quadrant values for each service line or department are plugged into the equation and a total value is calculated for each line by multiplying the quadrant value by the weight of 0.2. Again, this becomes the starting point for discussion, and although not as visually appealing or readily illuminating as a portfolio matrix or graph, it enables the organization to include an unlimited number of variables in the overall equation.

The third and most sophisticated analysis entails a risk coefficient, much like that used in evaluating investment strategies (sometimes termed a beta coefficient). This is included for those executives or board members who may be reluctant (perhaps rightfully so) to discard or diminish a particular service line or department. This method attempts to quantify the downside of taking dramatic action on particular subcomponents of the organization's portfolio. This is a highly subjective calculation. Nonetheless, if nothing else, it offers individuals an opportunity to voice their opinions, air their concerns, and attempt to assess the fall-out of proposed actions. Such fall-out could include physician disquietude, media criticism, community disgruntlement, political response, or a diminishment of employee morale. An added consideration is that of competitor reaction and overall market consequences.

The risk coefficient can be developed in a number of ways — some of them very sophisticated models developed by consultants, academicians, or planning gurus. A rather simple yet effective starting point can be the same numerical assignment to each variable, as mentioned above. In this situation, however, the "reaction" of each group, organization, or constituency can be assigned a numerical value in terms of the overall impact on the hospital or health system considering the action. The risk coefficient becomes a diminishing number (a fraction or decimal) that reduces the overall value of the figure calculated above.

For example, the variable of "publicity" can be given ranking on a scale of decimals based on the expected degree of negative publicity that might offset the favorable financial impact of dropping a service line. The same approach can be used for political response, physician disquietude, and so forth.

By assigning a numerical value to some of these typically nonquantitative variables (or consequences), the executives and board considering such actions not only open up the dialogue for discussing the downside, they provide a more objective format for evaluating the likely impact. Since the assignment of numerical values is admittedly objective, arriving at an agreed-upon value will be a challenge and is not likely to be readily achieved through consensus. One suggestion is to use some kind of group average or Delphi method (in which everyone assigns his or her value anonymously) to facilitate the process to avoid boardroom brawls or long-hour impasses.

The actual method or process for arriving at such a determination is not nearly as important as the exercise in conducting the evaluation. As stated earlier, this is the most sophisticated method of analysis. However, if such risk analysis of possible consequences had been seriously evaluated by other organizations and other industries (e.g., Firestone and Ford in the case of the Explorer debacle), great expense and tragedy may have been averted.

6. Develop Annual Service Line Business Plans
Tied to the Budget Process

After the initial strategy is laid out and the plans are understood and virtually carved in tablets of stone, the ongoing evaluation is essential. To accomplish this, the organization must establish the notion of service line management as pervasive. It should not be considered a one-time attempt or a once-a-year activity. Rather, it should become an integral component of operating discussion, evaluation, and consideration. The concept and its applications should be known throughout the entire organization, noted, and promoted by senior management as a mainstay of the organization.

This can be accomplished in a variety of ways, the most effective of which is to periodically highlight the accomplishments of the service line managers and their teams. This is done in other industries that operate strategic business units, so it should not be difficult to replicate in healthcare. Awards could be given to the teams that achieve their goals and provide great value to the organization. This occurs already for many departments in hospitals and healthcare organizations. The difference is that it is more multidisciplinary in focus for the team and thus should serve to cross-pollinate success and camaraderie among various departments.

An inherent component of an effective service line setup is the integration of individual service line plans into the overall business or strategic plan of the organization. This should align with the budgeting process and should be symbiotic with all the planning timetables and documents. Here, a symbiosis would represent a balance between what the service lines are expected to do and what the organization needs to do.

The service line plans should fold into the organizational business plan on an annual basis and be driven by the strategic plan that the system has developed for its three- to five-year horizon. As with any truly effective business plan, the service line plans should be dynamic and fluid. The plans should be updated often enough to reflect the changing conditions in the market and assess topical opportunities as well as imminent threats.

7. As the Process Takes Root, Gradually Incorporate Other Departments and Areas

Early in this discussion I mentioned the danger of starting out with too many areas or too vast a number of service lines, especially those that cannot be readily measured. However, as the process gains awareness, establishes credibility, and improves performance, management may want to consider adding other service lines and eventually those areas that are not as easily classified with standard data. This should be considered only after a few years of operational acclimation with the more traditional service lines.

The rationale for eventually broadening the application to other areas of the hospital or health system is twofold. First, it provides some reassurance at the outset of the process that every area will have its day, so that critical department managers or directors do not feel they are left out of an important systemwide initiative. Second, it reinforces the validity and opportunity of the service line concept as a management tool designed to optimize organizational resources and ensure market competitiveness.

SUMMARY OF THE STEPS TO STREAMLINING

- Embrace the attitude that svelte is better.
- Develop the criteria for evaluating service lines.

- Assign service line managers to each line.
- Conduct a service line audit and array the lines by evaluative criteria.
- Determine strategy as an organization.
- Develop annual service line business plans tied into the budget process.
- As the process takes root, gradually incorporate other departments and areas.

This discussion should serve to underscore the inherent value in service line analysis and a commitment to streamline operations, which is the discipline of ongoing evaluation on a "business unit" basis. This analysis or evaluation represents the primary missing component and separates (not in a favorable way) healthcare from the bulk of American industry. Most other enterprises within the American system place great stock in and managerial stewardship on their ability to subdivide their businesses by strategic business units (SBUs). This subdivision enables them to weed out the underperformers, or at least target them for consolidation, focused effort, or resource reduction, and concentrate on the organizational "stars" that offer greater prospects for expansion and opportunity for sustaining the core. In that regard, as an industry healthcare would be well served to learn a lesson from our industrial counterparts and enterprising colleagues.

NOTES

1. Portions of this chapter were previously published in the *Journal of Healthcare Management.*

2. Many articles exist on service line management and can be traced via the Internet or through healthcare marketing trade groups and associations. The first definitive book on the subject was *Product Management for Hospitals: Organizing for Profitability* (Folger and Gee 1987).

REFERENCES

Folger, J., and E. P. Gee. 1987. *Product Management for Hospitals: Organizing for Profitability.* Chicago: American Hospital Association.

Healthcare Advisory Board. 1999. *The Physician Perspective: Key Drivers of Physician Loyalty.* Research Findings from the 1998 National Survey and Conjoint Analysis. Washington, DC: The Advisory Board Company.

2

Use the Internet as a Management Tool[1]

The Internet is your business.

—Michael Dell

WHEN CONSIDERING STRATEGIES for improving hospital and health system margins, the Internet is arguably the best option for the long term. This chapter is placed toward the front of the book for two reasons. First, healthcare is excruciatingly and inexplicably behind most of American industry in applying the Internet, so we have no time for delay. Second, an effective Web-based strategy can, and should, form the foundation for the remaining strategies that will be outlined in the ensuing chapters.

The Internet is *not* just a marketing strategy, nor is it fundamentally promotional, educational, or informational. It is, as the above quote from Michael Dell states, *the* way of doing business in the information age. Yet the reality is that many hospital and health system CEOs probably still regard the Internet as little more than an "electronic brochure." Such reasoning is not only seriously flawed, it is debilitating because that kind of mental model will either delay or defer altogether the rapid deployment of the Internet as a pivotal tool for managing healthcare in the third millennium. The thrust of this chapter is to make the argument for a concerted effort to embrace the Net as a fundamental, if not essential, forum for conducting business. In other words, I suggest making Web-based healthcare delivery a *very* high priority.

THE NEW IDS

The first move in embracing the use of the Net as an organizational model and an operational tool is to recognize that the healthcare industry needs to rethink its long-standing position. For the past few years, many have believed that organizational viability hinged on developing an effective integrated delivery system (IDS). The hard lesson learned during that time is that the IDS model makes for great theory and good business for consultants, but it does not result in a better configuration or a more competitive health system—either at the local level or on the national front.

Therefore, given the drift (one might call it a tidal wave) of American industry to Web-based technology, healthcare leaders should consider a new IDS, namely an integrated *digital* system. Although many are still skeptical of the power and potential of the Internet (especially in the wake of the resounding crash of so many dot-com firms), the fact remains that this force is changing the way we do business and conduct our personal affairs. For this industry and for individual organizations, it realistically offers a potential escape hatch from the crashing wave of market turbulence and the subsequent pressure on the bottom line. Although it may be too premature to guarantee economic salvation from this new communication forum, extensive data in other industries and preliminary data within our own support the claim that efficiencies may be gained and a competitive advantage achieved.

TANGIBLE SAVINGS FROM THE INTERNET

Just how real is the potential and how vast the savings? According to a report by SunTrust Equitable Securities Corporation, healthcare "represents the single most attractive growth opportunity on the Internet today, with over $250 billion in administrative and redundant costs waiting to be streamlined" (Morrissey 1999). That number represents a practically inconceivable dollar amount at a global level, let alone a local application. Yet a few empirical examples already support the value of Internet initiatives.

A group of four doctors in New Hampshire realized net savings of over $120,000 annually by implementing electronic medical records. A hospital in Seattle saved eight dollars in staff cost for each Web referral it received (Healthcare Advisory Board 1999). And an article in *Managed Care* estimated that the cost of filing a hospital insurance claim can drop to as little as five cents per transaction through the Net compared with $1.25 for a paper claim and 25 cents through conventional data interchange. This coincides with data from the financial services industry, which has seen costs drop from $1.35 with a bank teller to ten cents on the Net (Pedersen 1999). The bottom line in both a literal and figurative sense is that sizeable savings in transaction costs may be had—and that represents just one facet of operation.

Tremendous savings may be realized in several areas of Internet application; an obvious one is that of administrative or back-office functions. As with other industries that have successfully adopted and embraced Internet applications, a significant degree of inherent inefficiency exists in service industries that can be reduced, if not eliminated, via this communication and access tool. Opportunities exist in other areas of critical hospital operation, such as revenue cycle management, which could involve online payment by consumers as well as links to payers. Several initiatives are under way for supply chain purchasing and administration. This actually has proven to be one of the most successful and readily adopted means of improving efficiency, whether through online inventory management or by facilitating and improving the entire procurement process. Care and case management is another avenue that is being explored by progressive organizations throughout the country. This includes everything from disease management to wireless medication administration.

SHIFTING RESPONSIBILITY TO THE CUSTOMER

At its core, the Internet shifts the work responsibility from an organization representative to the consumer (or patient, patient's family, doctor, and so forth) or another involved party. Consider the commonplace example of scheduling airline reservations. Under the traditional mode of scheduling a reservation, the airline would (by necessity) employ someone—even if a travel agent was involved—to take the information, process the reservation, and mail out the confirmation, either in the form of a ticket or an itinerary for electronic ticketing. The Internet automates most, if not all, of those functions and places the work flow responsibility squarely on the shoulders of the consumer. Yet the consumer clearly does not appear to mind assuming the responsibility or incurring the additional workload, as the process is usually more time efficient than the traditional method.

In essence, the Internet is all about "disintermediation"—eliminating the intermediary in the transaction. All this may seem patently obvious, yet many healthcare executives fail to see the value of the medium even when they understand its fundamental role. If more healthcare managers considered how many transactions occur within the healthcare exchange, they might get more excited about the breadth of possibilities available through this tool.

Skeptics will argue—and many do—that healthcare is different. It is too individualized and too compassionate for something as impersonal and intangible as the Internet. That argument may make for a maudlin excuse, but it is neither reasonable nor representative of how patients and other customers of the healthcare delivery system feel. Ask patients who have had to supply the same information to four different admissions clerks during the course of their hospital experience and you will find that the experience was not necessarily personal, caring, or compassionate. Rather, it seems fundamentally redundant, inefficient, and archaic. Much of the population wonders why this industry, which seems so impressively advanced in terms of medical discoveries and scientific technology, can be so backward in its adoption of information technology and application of electronic communication.

OTHER CONSIDERATIONS BEYOND FINANCIAL

In addition to the cost side of the equation, all-important considerations exist on the customer side. A sophisticated Web-based network not only makes referrals and transfer of information for physicians more efficient, it links doctors in ways that are legally acceptable (as opposed to some financial arrangements) and organizationally efficient.

Great opportunities also abound for building patient networks that are loyalty producing. As with other Web-based industries and companies, the Net provides the means by which patients (or customers) can more readily access the system and more efficiently utilize its resources.

Finally, the Internet offers an invaluable communication and evaluation tool in dealing with payers and purchasers. Insurance companies are, for the most part, more advanced than health systems in using the Net, but they still must rely on providers for the two-way communication flow. At the same time, employers welcome a pervasive application of the Net, especially as they consider different intermediary strategies such as defined contribution or organizing employer coalitions.

Although the Net is admittedly not a panacea for all the challenges facing our industry, it is one of the best avenues for improving organizational efficiency and achieving sustainable cost reduction. At the same time, it is the accepted and expected mechanism for aligning customer interests and information with provider resources. It is vital to local healthcare providers to get up to speed on the Net. If we do not, we run the risk of losing our preeminent position as the source for health-related information and healthcare delivery.

SEVEN STEPS TO UTILIZING THE INTERNET
AS A MANAGEMENT TOOL

1. Get the CEO to Champion the Initiative

Making utilization of the Net an operational imperative in healthcare is for some organizations quite problematic, if not implausible. Chief among the reasons for this is the reluctance, recalcitrance, or outright skepticism of the chief executive officer. At a recent conference on Internet applications in healthcare, one of the leading figures in the industry, a past chairman of the AHA, noted to someone in the hall, "This is fascinating stuff, but I have no idea what they're talking about" (author observation). That candid statement is a good summary of where many veteran healthcare executives stand when it comes to applying the Internet. Some experience a cognitive motor function disconnect when trying to understand and use the Internet as a tool; it is viewed as a radical alteration of the way we do business. To paraphrase an old saying, what we do not understand, we are not likely to embrace.

In simplest terms, some CEOs are not comfortable accessing the Internet. Consequently, they may be reluctant or ambivalent regarding committing significant resources to its application for their organization. In short, they are not likely to take their organization for a swim in waters in which they themselves rarely wade.

Hospital CEOs Out of Sync. Although this depiction may seem provincial and even archaic in a world where the Internet is viewed as essential for basic survival as the telephone once was, it is a harsh reality in healthcare. One survey finding that illustrated the disparity between other American industries and healthcare found that among CEOs of global concerns, 72 percent had "extremely active" or "moderately active" efforts in their Internet planning and strategy initiatives. Another 8 percent had "somewhat active" efforts, with only 20 percent of those polled stating they had planned "no efforts" to incorporate Internet applications. Those results contrasted sharply with findings among hospital executives, where 73 percent of those surveyed stated they had "no e-strategy," leaving only 27 percent, or just over one-fourth, who went on record as having an e-strategy (H-Works 2001).

Therefore, as with most initiatives, the first step is to assess the CEO's interest in and comfort with the Internet. It may take some creativity to get the CEO motivated to commit major resources to this initiative, but ultimately it will be necessary. The organization that does not have the full support of the CEO and the involvement of its board will be subject to constant review and justification of the resources required in making the Net an integral part of its operating strategy. Furthermore, when the budgets tighten, a natural gravitational pull will ensue to diminish, detour from, or discard altogether Internet initiatives. The progressive and successful healthcare system cannot let that happen. The CEO must not only be sold on the need for the Internet, he or she needs to be an advocate and a champion, driving the process and monitoring its planning, development, and successful execution. One of the most recognized and highly regarded CEOs in the United States, Jack Welch, exemplifies an invaluable lesson to be learned from American enterprise: he was the person responsible for integrating the Net into the operations of the world's largest company, General Electric. The situation is not all that different for a freestanding hospital or a major healthcare system. The CEO must be fully engaged, completely supportive, and intensely involved in operationalizing the Internet for it to ever have a reasonable chance of optimizing its capabilities and transforming the organization.

2. Incorporate the Internet and IT into the Strategic Plan

Few things motivate hospital executives like the proposition of losing ground in the market or sustaining serious financial losses. Although many executives know well that they should be playing in the Internet sandbox, they probably do not see such activity as crucial to their very professional existence. So, the challenge and charge to the organization that has a CEO who has embraced the need for the Net is this: make it integral to operations, persuading senior management and other individuals in key leadership roles that information technology is not a silo strategy. Rather, it is an integral part of the organization's body politic.

As time goes on, this may not be a difficult case to make. Right now, as mentioned earlier, relatively few hospitals and health systems are actively pursuing e-strategy. Among those, a much smaller percentage of systems and hospitals have committed significant money and resources to taking advantage of the Internet. Some of these efforts have been well publicized, but because they are so few in number, too many executives may still be rationalizing that these are what are known in marketing parlance as innovators or perhaps early adopters. Consequently, executive teams that are too comfortable, complacent, or conservative may put off an Internet strategy until "the next phase" of its implementation. The rationale behind this sentiment is that so many of these innovators and early adopters get burned and lose their shirts, or even their jobs, by bolting out of the blocks too early.

This reluctance is understandable in light of the unfortunate experiences that many healthcare managers have had with inefficient and ineffective information systems. If you want to see a healthcare executive's temperature rise, ask him or her about some of the money they have poured down the drain on information systems—hardware and software that has gotten them nowhere.

Organizations that Hesitate Are Lost. Although such hesitation is understandable, even defensible, the problem with that "wait-until-the-next-phase" logic is indigenous to the Internet itself, namely the concept of rapid change and lightning speed. Organizations in other industries that have banked on second-wave development and adoption have found themselves haplessly stranded on the shore, losing ground and market share to competitors who caught the first wave and adapted to the advanced technology.

Hospitals will likely find themselves in this condition. Of course, some role will always exist for even the latest adopters of the Internet, but they will lose so much ground on the learning curve and on the basic applications that by the time they decide to play, the game will largely be decided.

The economic pundits and Wall Street analysts may finally have their say in this area of healthcare regarding rapid implementation, economies of scale and scope, and the ability to capture accompanying market share. In other words, the Internet may be an arena in which the principles of business and commerce *actually work*, unlike so many other previous times when they have not.

Hospitals and Health Systems that Are Leading the Charge. Kaiser has committed approximately $2 billion to the Internet. Sharp Healthcare, a prestigious organization in Southern California, has committed many people and considerable resources to the initiative. Duke University Medical Center has devoted extensive monetary investment and resources to the Net. Perhaps the executives at Kaiser, Sharp, Duke, and other progressive organizations have read the literature on the potential savings that can accrue to organizations that incorporate the infrastructure and operational abilities of the Net. And perhaps they have spent a fair amount of time and resources on consultants who tell them how to get a major step ahead of their competition. In so doing, they become the first and the fastest to bring the technology of the Internet to bear on the delivery of healthcare.

Consider what HCA–the Healthcare Company (formerly known as Columbia) is doing. Purportedly, one of HCA's senior executives once quipped (admittedly during the height of the dot-com frenzy), "I never knew I'd be working for an Internet company that just happens to own hospitals." That comment was obviously lighthearted and exaggerated, but the fact remains that for its first few years following the transition from its turbulent days as Columbia to the reconfigured, remodeled, and reconstituted HCA, this company had left its web site operations on autopilot. Yet, in the summer of 1999, under the direction of the company's president, HCA made a corporate commitment to get all its hospitals online with its web site department, eHC. In making that commitment, which at the time seemed to be nothing less than a Herculean feat, the nation's largest healthcare company gave notice to the industry that it would not be left behind in the realm of information technology and electronic communication. Consequently, the giant hospital company successfully brought 140 of its more than 200 hospitals online in just over a year; now the entire firm is "wired." That includes everything from sophisticated health systems with existing sites to smaller facilities that had never before seen a web site in their dreams.

These are a few, but nonetheless prominent, examples of health systems that have decided that the Internet would become a major part of their operation strategy and an integral part of their forward planning. Other hospitals and health systems should take their cue from them and follow their lead. The initiative needs to become an integral part of the strategy, not a separate silo that only occasionally gets attention and capital. It can be neither a promotion-only function that belongs in the realm of the marketing department nor an information systems–driven endeavor that is primarily the purview of the technologically gifted. It needs to be as integral to the organization's strategy as the budgeting process — or at least a close second.

To accomplish this, a few tactical considerations and steps will ensure a more ready assimilation of the Internet and IT into the overall strategy of the system. The first requires the chief information officer (CIO; assuming the organization has one) to become part of the senior management team. From this easily implemented tactic, management can ensure that IT strategy is part of every initiative the organization pursues. Rather than have a separate strategy, IT and the Internet should be woven into the fabric of every strategy.

3. Review Other Models Within and Outside the Industry

One suggestion that will save a great deal of money, energy, and frustration is to tap into the experience of other organizations that have paved the path for those coming later to the technology. This does not have to be restricted to organizations within the healthcare milieu, as much can be gleaned from enterprises outside the industry in terms of creative applications and avoidable pitfalls. Historically, healthcare organizations have not proven very adept at adopting the practices and protocols of companies outside the industry. This is unfortunate, especially in the realm of the Internet, because many industries and the firms within them have been effectively utilizing it for several years. Since many of the functions applicable to and affected by the Internet are administrative and nonclinical, a great deal of crossover can be seen in similar applications.

Not a long time ago, the interested hospital or health system would have had to go outside the industry to regard a functioning Internet application and system. However, within the past two or three years several leading players have, as mentioned above, committed sizeable resources and considerable time to incorporating Internet strategies into their long-range operational configuration and business plans. A few of these systems are quite prominent and therefore spotlighted in the news. Some have gone so far as to offer their experience as a prototype—a few out of the collegiality of the profession, and a few for a consulting fee. A field trip to one of these facilities is probably well worth the time and any money required.

In addition, some consulting firms spotlight and chronicle the best-practices hospitals and health systems. These third-party advisors can help a system jump-start its effort and ensure that the organization gets off to the right start with adequate commitment and sufficient understanding. Such firms may be worth their consulting fee if they are able to translate the formula for success from best-practices hospitals into a language and operating style that will work for their clients. Not all of the firms that claim the ability to do so are successful, but even if they accomplish a fraction of what they promise, they are probably worth the expense.

Major Money, Little Sense. Some hospitals and health systems have proven to be penny-wise and pound-foolish in this regard. They have spent millions of dollars on high tech hardware and state-of-the-art software but have been miserly when hiring experts on the implementation side. Questioning why the magnificent boxes with the marvelous software will not perform for them, many executives have experienced mounting frustration regarding IT solutions. They have expected their existing internal staff to take highly sophisticated, complex equipment and work wonders with minimal resources and insufficient skill sets. When it fails to accomplish the tasks for which it was purchased, the executives either blame their hapless employees or curse the vendor who sold it to them. They have difficulty seeing the error of their ways and the faulty repetition of their style.

One way to avoid this kind of frugality failure is to work with a team from a pioneering health system or a consulting group that has proven itself with a wide range of clients. This area is quite foreign to many well-meaning but ill-trained and poorly equipped hospital staff, and precious little time is available for on-the-job training and off-the-record mistakes. The bottom line is, better to pony up and pay for the people who can ensure a successful execution than to have the latest and greatest but not know how to use it.

4. Enlist Outside Design Assistance

One of the blessings and curses of the healthcare industry in the United States is that it derives from the expert model construct. That is a boon to the industry because the industry drivers —

physicians—are undoubtedly the best trained, most highly educated, most thoroughly equipped medical practitioners in the world. They are experts in their profession and outstanding in their field.

Problems with the Expert Model. The expert model is by contrast the bane of American enterprise as it is patronizing, out of sync with the market, and antiquated. American enterprise pivots on the buyer; it is market driven and consumer oriented. In many ways it is the antithesis of the expert model, assuming that the consumer is the expert and therefore the driver of change and dictator of direction. In this model, however, myriad "dictators" vote with their feet and rule with their pocketbook. It is, quite simply, the most efficient form of economic exchange structure in the history of the world.

Then there is healthcare. As a corporate director of human resources for a Fortune 100 firm said, "Healthcare is the last bastion of inefficiency in the United States." This statement gives one very good reason for enlisting "outsiders" in the design of the Internet. The Internet is the archetype of the "democratic dictatorship" that is the American market enterprise. The Internet allows freedom of thought movement throughout the world and allows its user to select the sites and the messages that appeal uniquely to his or her taste. Based on that dynamic, organizations that fail to enlist not only input but specific design specifications on their Internet offerings will fail. It is that simple.

Audiences to Poll. Hospitals and health systems need to consider and consult with a variety of audiences. One of the most important is the at-large consumer, who may one day become the in-house patient. Consumers who surf the Web are not much different from consumers who shop at malls because the Internet has become so pervasive (up to 90 million Americans use it) that it cuts across every category of individual in the nation. Even older citizens, who were once thought to be too engrained, too afraid, or too ambivalent to use the Internet, now represent one of its most rapidly growing demographic sectors. Developing a configuration and an orientation that meets the needs of consumers should not be difficult, as "product testers" are everywhere.

Another key audience that should be consulted prior to casting the Net is the medical staff. As mentioned earlier, the Internet is a tremendous vehicle for increasing the loyalty of physicians and bonding them to a hospital or health system. Make the doctor's life easier and he or she will make the administrator's life happier. At a recent conference in Chicago on Internet applications, an orthopedic surgeon recounted how the hospital where he practices had made radiological scans available over the Internet so that he was able to view them without having to come down to the ER. He recited an anecdote in which he was at home watching a movie with his kids one Friday evening when he received two calls from the ER that would normally have required him to leave home and go to the hospital. In both instances he was able to view the scans on his home computer. He then called the ER staff to inform them that the patients involved in the accidents—who, by coincidence, were both neighbors of the doctor—did not have broken bones and that he could see them in his office the next day. He concluded by asking the room full of hospital CEOs, "Now do you think I am going to even think about referring or admitting any of my patients to another hospital than that one?"

With respect to physician relations, the Internet could be termed the *killer application/super glue*. However, just providing the service does not endear physicians. There is no guarantee that "if you offer it, they will surf." In fact, some systems have failed so miserably to enlist the physicians in the design of the Web applications that they have alienated the physicians. In one case, the hospital's system was so inefficient and ineffectual related to one doctor's ability to access from his home computer that he quipped, "It would be faster for me to drive to the ER than to try to bring up the record on my computer from home" (H-Works 2001).

Do Not Disregard Employers. Another important audience that merits attention and should provide feedback is the employer group. This group is often overlooked, if not ignored altogether, by healthcare executives. Yet this influential stakeholder group accounts for a large share of the care purchased and an increasing amount of decisions made. Employers become even more relevant as the delivery system moves toward more consumerism with greater accountability and individual decision making. The consumerism movement flows perfectly with the enormous increase in Internet use, as employees are now able to more readily access information from competing health plans and choose a plan that meets their individual needs or those of their family. This movement, which has gained considerable momentum within the past two years, has spawned an entire new sector in healthcare, one that bypasses the insurance brokers and theoretically eliminates middle-man costs while enabling and empowering the employee. Companies such as Vivius have attracted both media attention and venture capital in their attempt to give consumers more control over their decisions and employers less administrative hassle (and perhaps even reduced costs).

In addition, the very trend to provide more services on the Net is consistent with the trend toward consumerism that is rising in the healthcare industry. We are an industry in transition, and nowhere is this more manifest than in the milieu of the Internet. The fact remains that people expect the Internet to be a ready source for healthcare information access. It follows, then, that the Net would be a likely vehicle for healthcare transactions of all types. The big question for many Web-savvy consumers is why our industry has taken so long to even start to incorporate practices that have been in place in other industries (e.g., finance, transportation, entertainment) for more than five years.

5. Start Small, Build Gradually, and Begin with the End in Mind

One of the biggest mistakes organizations make in approaching the Internet is trying to do too much too quickly—in essence, to consume the elephant in one meal. Such a flawed approach only leads to frenzy, frustration, and eventual abandonment of the initiative. Although that may seem like a blinding flash of the obvious, a surprising number of organizations make that egregious error.

First, when healthcare executives finally do realize how relevant the Net is, and how far behind they are, they can easily lapse into panic. In an effort to catch up, they may try to accomplish too much with far too little capability. It is reminiscent of the Midwest hospital executive who had an epiphany regarding Y2K preparations at a conference in November of 1999. He came back from the conference and nearly drove his staff crazy and his hospital into the ground in his eleventh hour attempt to make up for lost time.

Urgency, Not Panic. Although a sense of urgency is necessary when embracing and incorporating information technology, there should never be a sense of panic, as this will ultimately kill the effort and alienate many people in the process. Additionally, reactive resolutions and panic-driven directives are usually poorly planned, insufficiently financed, and thus eventually destined to falter and fail. Taking the time to start small and gradually build on the initial development is a far better course.

Part of the problem with starting small is knowing where to start, as so much often needs to be done just to catch up. Deciding where the most important entrance is can be a maddening exercise in itself. This is where a consultant or an organizational mentor can help. However, in the case of the latter, the lagging organization must be cautious not to exactly mirror the implementation schedule and project prioritization of the mentoring hospital, as their market conditions may be quite different from the experienced hospital.

Identify Early Wins. An old managerial maxim states that "when confronted with major multiple tasks that require considerable capital and commitment, start with some early, easy victories." Along that line of thinking, an assistant CIO at a leading Internet-advanced system in the upper Midwest advised attendees at an Internet applications conference to consider electronic signature for physicians. Based on his experience, this was a relatively easy procedure to implement with minimal expenditure and sizeable dividends. For that particular hospital, it secured the loyalty of many "splitting" physicians.

That is a good pattern to follow at the outset. Pick some small, relatively simple wins and build on them. However, rather than just launching with an Internet strategy that looks like a patchwork quilt, the organization must begin the initiative with an overall plan for implementation. In essence, the organization should map out where the initiative is going and what the end product will look like in three to five years, or whatever time horizon it chooses. This leads to discussion of another fundamental mistake that many organizations commit in their Internet strategy: They just start building a presence, rather than establishing what that presence will eventually look like when they're finished.

This ties back to step 2, the need for integrating the Internet initiative into the overall strategic plan. If that is done thoroughly and successfully, the process will force a clear definition of what the Web-based services look like and accomplish several years down the road.

6. Make the Internet Pervasive Throughout the Organization

After specifying each of the prior steps, the Internet should have a pervasive presence throughout the entire organization. Management at Dell Computer has done just this. In essence, they have infused in their staff the sense that the Net is their vehicle for conducting business—internally and externally. Although we may be a fair distance from that kind of cultural phenomenon in healthcare, progressive organizations will likely see that as a desired objective in the next few years. Again, we should not anticipate that the compassionate component of healthcare will be replaced by the insensitive and impersonal sense of high tech but rather augmented by what the technology can do to improve outcomes and increase face time with caregivers. The organizations within the industry that are aggressively pursuing the rapid deployment of information technology understand this fundamental precept and are attempting to move their entire organization along this road, not just the managers, staff personnel, and administrative departments.

The Importance of Internal Education. To effectively transition from the former style of minimal IT and create an organization that is strategically wired and emphatically personal requires a great deal of education and information. Many people in this industry—from those who serve on the front lines to those who work in the back office—have deep-seated concerns about the impact of technology on their professions and their personal careers. Healthcare executives should not expect the vast number of people affected by their opinions and their interaction to spontaneously or even eventually understand the role of technology. They need to see the big picture as well as understand the small print when considering information technology—in essence, to be given the same kind of vision and sense of direction that the managerial team receives in the process of accepting the concept in the first place. They need to clearly understand how this new wave of technology will allow them to be better employees and their organization a better place at which to work and provide a more conducive environment in which to be cared for.

That understanding and sense of vision and direction should permeate the organization. This will lead to less resistance and more support, as well as fewer concerns and greater enthusiasm for facilitating the adoption and incorporation of the Internet as an organizationwide instrument for improving the quality of care and increasing the caliber of employees.

Creating this type of environment can be accomplished via a number of avenues and a variety of media, from the employee newsletter to CEO town hall meetings. Of course, the avenue of the Internet itself may be utilized, but managers should not assume that this would be the best medium to communicate the effectiveness of it. And executives should also be careful to not alienate those who are technophobic or passively aggressively nostalgic. This can be a frightening technology and a frustrating transition; managers should set the tone by being patient and realistic.

7. *Never Become Stagnant with the Endeavor*

The Internet is known for its speed. The fitting title of Bill Gates's book captures the essence of the computer age, *Business at the Speed of Thought*. Correspondingly, organizations must be vigilant in their constant pursuit of ways to upgrade their technology and improve and modify their strategy and presence. This is a very different approach for an industry known for traditional practices and long-standing policies. However, a measured pace in terms of the Internet and information technology is the equivalent of yesterday's news.

To that extent, several of the prior steps should be considered on an ongoing basis, such as engaging consultants, seeking guidance from mentoring organizations, enlisting the design expertise and advice of customers, and constantly updating the strategic plan to reflect the latest developments and to consider future ramifications in the IT world.

In that regard, the Internet and the pervasive application of information technology may be just the boost this industry needs to keep us *au courant,* relevant, and viable. If it achieves that alone, it is well worth all the money expended on the endeavor.

SUMMARY OF THE STEPS TO MAKING THE INTERNET A MANAGEMENT TOOL

- Get the CEO to champion the initiative.
- Incorporate the Internet and IT into the strategic plan.
- Review other models within and outside the industry.
- Enlist outside design assistance.
- Start small, build gradually, and begin with the end in mind.
- Make the Internet pervasive throughout the organization.
- Never become stagnant with the endeavor.

When Ronald Reagan was president and before the Berlin Wall came down in 1989, he made reference to the United States as the "last, best hope for democracy in the world." In retrospect, perhaps he was not far off. Similarly, although not nearly as globally grandiose nor historically significant, the Internet may be this industry's last, best hope for preserving the healthcare system we are accustomed to and comfortable with.

The nation's health system is probably in its most precarious position in decades, if not ever. Articles and editorials started appearing by the fall of 2000 that questioned whether the mas-

sive and pervasive problems the nation's system faces could ever
be resolved. As employers face yet another year of dramatic
increases in their healthcare premiums and Americans look forward to increased deductibles, higher copayments, and less dis-
cretionary income, the nation's policymakers seem reticent to, if
not incapable of, developing plans to resolve the issue. Having
witnessed the Great Clinton Health Plan Bonfire, most politicians are highly reluctant to stick their necks out to make proposals, let alone specific plans. In essence, as pundits and politicians
point out, we are faced now with the same situation as in 1992,
with no relief for the nation's ills visible for the immediate or
long-term future.

Managed care has run its course—both in terms of concentration of the market (it is now on the decline in terms of
number of enrollees) and cost control. The savings have been
realized, and we are now in a recovery and recouping mode.
Americans do not like the idea of restricted access to care and
yet do not want to shoulder the burden of increasing costs that
accompany unlimited access. We also want the latest and the
best that technology has to offer; yet this comes with a price—a
high one.

Why Not Actually Bring Down Costs?

We appear to be caught in a loop regarding cost. As with most
situations that appear to have no rational means of resolution,
the situation reaches a climax and the proposed solutions are
politically expedient, operationally reactive, and financially dev-
astating. That will probably be the case with the nation's healthcare system as well, unless we find a way to bring the costs under
control. The big problem is that we have no way to bring costs
under control. The only time in recent American history that
such a phenomenon has occurred was during the mid-1990s,
when the managed care companies were setting artificial pricing lower than costs to obtain market share. They will not do

that again, as they have learned that losing share is better than losing money: a smaller, profitable business is preferable to a large loser.

In the sense that healthcare is not experiencing declining costs and increased productivity, our industry is out of sync with other industries in the United States. Nearly every other business is showing dramatic increases in productivity and efficiency, but healthcare plods along like a 1950 Chevy, guzzling gas and costing the nation more than it wants to pay for the slow ride. The main difference between our industry and others is the failure to adopt the latest in information technology, where many of the gains are being achieved in American industry other than healthcare.

Walking into a hospital (in most cases), you will experience the same mode of operation that you would have experienced two decades ago. Name another industry in which that operational time warp exists. From an operational efficiency standpoint, healthcare is a dinosaur. The only reason we are not extinct and thus relegated to the Smithsonian Institution is that no viable option exists. But that will change in time—in a very short time. Whenever a commercial void appears and customer discontent ensues, competition rises to the occasion. Healthcare is no exception, and the unforeseen, yet more efficient model waits in the wings.

The situation does not have to be dire. Information technology presents reasonable alternatives to bringing us out of the Neanderthal Age, and many of the applications involve the Internet. In a sense, when hospital CEOs and system executives embrace the Internet as their top priority, they are rendering a great service to the community and assisting their industry in moving into the information age. In so doing, they become not only good citizens, but keepers of the trust. Now is the time for every good CEO to come to the aid of his colleagues and advance the IT battle front to the next line.

NOTE

1. Portions of this chapter were previously published in the *Journal of Healthcare Management.*

REFERENCES

Healthcare Advisory Board. 1999. *Financial Impact of the Internet on Costs*, p. 3. Washington, DC: The Advisory Board Company.

H-Works. 2001. *Health Care in the Internet Age*, pp. 8, 27. Washington, DC: The Advisory Board Company.

Morrissey, J. 1999. "The Mouse is Roaring: Internet Technology Is Slashing the Time it Takes to Get Needed Data to and from Providers." *Modern Healthcare* 29 (32): 52–54, 56, 58.

Pedersen, D. 1999. "The Inevitability of E-Commerce." *Managed Care* June: 36–40.

3

Enhance the System Through Co-opetition[1]

A rising tide lifts all boats.

—John F. Kennedy

HEALTHCARE IS POISED and ready for the concept of co-opetition. Very possibly, co-opetition represents not only the next wave for the industry but a new era for the nation's largest service sector. On a fundamental level, co-opetition may offer the most feasible and immediate means to ensuring the survival of the industry as we know it. An industrywide collaborative approach that establishes uniform standards, common access, comparable benchmarks, and meaningful quality measures may be the best counteroffensive to the push for nationalized healthcare and federalized medicine.

DEFINITION AND EXAMPLES OF CO-OPETITION

Co-opetition is a relatively new term in American management, dating back to the early 1990s. Ray Norda, founder of Novell

53

Corporation, coined the term; it derives from combining the words "cooperation" and "competition." Co-opetition could be defined as the optimal blend of competition and cooperation. The notion behind this definition is that all organizations operating in a free-market environment must compete, yet at some times and with some projects, organized collaboration is the optimal avenue, offering the best outcome.

In 1996, academicians Adam Brandenburger of the Harvard Business School and Barry Nalebuff of the Yale School of Management wrote a best-selling book on the topic entitled, aptly, *Co-Opetition*. As they note, the concept has been applied in most industries and, most recently, effectively deployed in the information technology field, where it appears to have taken root and borne fruit (Brandenburger and Nalebuff 1996). Innovative companies like Intel and integrative concerns like Sematech have shown that co-opetition not only benefits individual organizations, it can improve the overall performance of an industry.

Co-opetition also differs from collaboration in its reach. One usually thinks of collaboration on a horizontal level (e.g., in our industry, hospital to hospital). For healthcare, that application could also be extended to vertical integration or cooperation (hospital with physician group or physician group with surgery center). Co-opetition considers the entire sphere of an organization's or industry's reach.

A case in point is found in Brandenburger and Nalebuff's book involving the auto industry. The situation depicted in this example occurred early in the history of automobiles, long before they were as pervasive as they are today. Two major automakers teamed up with a tire manufacturer and other auto parts suppliers on an initiative to encourage the development of more roadways throughout the country. Each of the participating organizations realized that the number of roadways not only limited capacity, it had a direct effect on the demand for automobiles. This co-opetive venture was very successful and laid the groundwork for the development of the U. S. interstate system.

Athough much has been written about co-opetition in other sectors of American industry, it is rarely mentioned in healthcare. A review of healthcare literature over the past five years produces only a handful of articles on the topic. These articles suggest that application of the concept has not only been minimal but somewhat isolated and project specific. The fact that healthcare executives have not embraced the concept is not surprising, given that the industry usually lags about five to ten years behind the high tech sector both in technology and in managerial theory and applications.

THE TIME IS RIGHT, COMPARABLE TO HIGH TECH

However, this industry is now at a juncture where collaborative ventures and cooperative attitudes may be both plausible and productive. In fact, healthcare may be just the industry in which co-opetition has the potential to function best. Certainly, many parallels are evident between the healthcare environment today and the high tech field in the late 1980s and early 1990s, when co-opetition proved to be a boon to that industry.

Like the high tech industry was at one point, healthcare is complex, balkanized, and locally differentiated. For many individuals, it can be difficult to access and easy to misunderstand.

These conditions lend themselves to co-opetive efforts to establish universal procedures, reduce complexity, increase understanding, and develop more user-friendly terminology and access. Furthermore, recent events and industrywide initiatives appear to indicate that our industry is moving toward a more

collaborative model, eschewing the combative attitude that sur-
faced during the early to mid-1990s. That hard-edge era of competition has hopefully taught us much about the nature of the
industry and the limits of competition.

THE UPSIDE AND DOWNSIDE OF COMPETITION

Competition within the healthcare industry is somewhat enig-
matic. It can be either boon or bane, depending on the attitude of the organization involved and the degree of competition.
Competition is a boon from the standpoint that the free-market
structure encourages innovation, fosters quality improvement,
and rewards efficiency. Despite recent rankings of healthcare
systems throughout the world (which placed the United States
37th), most would agree that the healthcare system in the United
States offers the highest quality, best outcomes, and most innovation. We can argue that our healthcare system leads the
world, both as the standard of quality and as the point of origin
for technology and improved medical treatment. Much of that
leadership can be attributed to the free-market underpinnings
on which our system is built.

This free-market architecture is also given credit for keeping
costs at an acceptable level. Admittedly, this latter argument
is currently under siege, given the double-digit insurance premium increases that many employers are experiencing. Nonetheless, the very notions of free enterprise with the inseparable
component of competition are proven pillars on which our current system rests.

One reason the notion of competitive markets is so attractive
is that the customer is the ultimate judge and jury. He or she will
base final judgment and selection on value factors, not capri-
cious or subjective criteria, thereby ensuring that "competitors"
will either meet the expectations of the market or suffer the
consequences.

However, the dark side of competition can emerge when local markets or national concerns shift from "friendly competition" to fierce aggression, or even combativeness. We can witness the results of this dynamic from the middle years of the 1990s, when combativeness in some markets produced vitriolic sentiments, media attacks, and expansion strategies—the equivalent of a medical arms race. We still encounter the aftermath of this period, which at times fostered duplicative services, exorbitant media expense, and illogical combinations. In retrospect, we observe that these tactics led to financial losses, shattered careers, physician disquietude, and public disenchantment.

In essence, we have observed that Jack Trammiel's oft-quoted maxim, "Business is war," does not apply to nor work well in the healthcare arena. The turbulent years of the 1990s prove that healthcare is a different organizational animal when considering fierce competition. Healthcare has always been more collaborative than other sectors of the nation's economy; collaboration is part of the healthcare DNA. For instance, the key operatives within healthcare, physicians, often work simultaneously at "competing hospitals," relying on similar technologies, procedures, and quality. This builds into the system a certain degree of cross-pollination of managerial techniques and operational standards.

Additionally, the nature of the field has historically been more collegial than other industries, with an educational framework and peer recognition component that more closely parallels the open-door atmosphere and collegiality of academia than the isolationist, clandestine attitude of more competitive industries. The very existence of the organization that published this book, the American College of Healthcare Executives (ACHE), is a prime example that educational advancement and collegial attitude are as much the mark of success in this industry as the market-based, monetary-oriented gauges of success so prominent in other industries.

In short, the "take-no-prisoners" attitude that is sometimes advanced in certain circles and seemingly rewarded in practical application does not lend itself congruently to healthcare. The years behind us clearly demonstrate that the public does not like it, politicians will not abide it, and the system will not absorb it. However, that does not mean we should get rid of competition altogether. To disrupt the existing mechanism and destroy the current model would be reactive and irrational. A better course would be to return to the days of more moderate competition, and an *even better* course would be to embrace the principles and practices of co-opetition.

COLLABORATIVE VENTURES AUGUR CO-OPETITION

Many indicators suggest we are entering an era when co-opetition may become a reality. On the national level, the formation of the Coalition to Protect America's Health Care is a fitting example and a meritorious effort on the part of its participants. This group involves many organizations, some of which were once fierce competitors. The goal of this collaborative venture is to educate the public and enlighten policymakers as to the critical need for financial and conceptual support for the nation's healthcare providers. This represents a groundbreaking effort and perhaps a bellwether initiative that signals a new day and a fresh approach to cooperation and collaboration within the industry.

This bodes well for the industry because collaboration is the essential first step in co-opetition. A spirit of collegiality is necessary, characterized by a willingness to sit down at the same table and work toward mutually beneficial solutions to industrywide problems. The difference between collaboration and co-opetition is not great, however: collaboration often involves a single issue, project, or concern. The outcome is usually a universally acceptable, episodically applicable solution that addresses that particular issue but does not fundamentally alter the basic mode of operation nor the delivery model under which the organizations function.

Theoretically, co-opetition moves beyond collaboration in addressing fundamental issues and problems. Examples in healthcare could range from the complexity of accessing the delivery system to the problematic rise in costs. These overarching issues are not only immense in scope, but seemingly insurmountable (in the near term) at the national level. However, as some markets have demonstrated, these types of issues can be addressed and improved in a relatively short time frame at a local level.

At the core of co-opetition is the idea that by improving the overall system at a level that is malleable and manageable, all parties benefit. Significantly, the party that benefits the most is the customer. And, as the technology industry has shown us in dramatic fashion, when the customer benefits, the entire sector benefits. In that sense, co-opetition is the practical application of President Kennedy's quote cited at the outset of this chapter. Co-opetition becomes the means to proactively and locally ensure that the tide moves in a favorable direction.

PROVEN ECONOMIC RESULTS OF COLLABORATION

As mentioned earlier, few examples of co-opetition are available in the industry. If they exist, they are not well publicized. However, one relatively recent study by the *Health Forum Journal* demonstrates that collaborative efforts are financially beneficial. The study cited a survey of 30 hospital CEOs, 25 of which reported that their hospitals had entered into collabo-

rative ventures that had resulted in savings from $300,000 to
$20 million (Coddington et al. 2000). These collaborative initia-
tives included services ranging from laundry services to imaging
centers. The study spotlights the inherent economic value of
collaborative efforts. For those who have worked in healthcare
for several years, such findings should not come as a surprise.

The nature of healthcare, despite being characterized as frac-
tionated, balkanized, disjointed (pick your adjective), provides
fertile ground to sow the seeds of collaboration. What other major sector in the United States still functions essentially as a
cottage industry? None come to mind because the inherent economics of cottage industries (i.e., localized organizations with
minimal regional or national affiliation) have become incom-
patible with the demands of the market and the desires of the
customers.

Yet, to a large extent, despite all the talk of mergers, ac-
quisitions, and consolidations, most hospitals remain local or
regional in their legal configuration. Certainly, national chains
exist—both for profit and not-for-profit—that are recognized for
their comparative size and their economic clout. Yet these larger
organzations still only represent a fraction of the total number
of hospitals. Compared to other major product and service industries, these larger companies are quite small in terms of the
proportion of the field they constitute. Of almost any major
industry—automobile, airline, computer hardware, accounting,
and so forth—four or five players represent over three-fourths
of the entire field. In healthcare, the largest organization in the
United States, HCA, controls less than 5 percent of the total number of hospitals in the nation. The top five national chains account for a combined total of less than one-fifth of the country's
hospitals. This is almost the exact inverse of most other major
industries in the United States, and yet healthcare remains the
largest service industry in the nation.

ACHIEVING LARGE-SCALE ECONOMIES
WITH FEWER PLAYERS

All of this means that the basic organizational structure of healthcare is out of sync with the American market model, which provides economies of scale, volume purchasing clout, and uniform operating practices. Yet the cottage-industry model remains intensely entrenched. Efforts to transform the industry to look more like its corporate cousins have largely been met with nominal success, if not outright failure, as shown by the current trend to disconnect or dismantle many of the couplings that occurred during the merger initiatives of the mid- to late 1990s.

Nonetheless, the economic advantages of large-scale organizations are relevant and perhaps even essential as the pressure intensifies on the delivery system to reign in costs and improve overall efficiency. Although some large-scale advantages can be achieved through national affiliations such as purchasing alliances, trade associations, or cooperatives, most of the major gains lie in local and regional ventures. In essence, this means partnering with the competition or teaming up with customers.

If significant savings can be achieved through collaborative ventures, imagine the realm of possibility for co-opetive initiatives that are more broad based and systemic. Co-opetition in its purest form involves more than just competitors—it includes "complementors," which for healthcare would mean payers, purchasers (employers or the government), and policymakers.

Fundamentally, co-opetition begins with dialogue and ends with redefinition. The target project can range from one as complex and comprehensive as redefining the access model to one more palatable and doable as simplifying the scheduling process. Whatever the initiative, the first step is to agree on a broad-based solution that cuts across industry sectors and market boundaries.

SEVEN STEPS TO ACHIEVING IMPROVED
PERFORMANCE THROUGH CO-OPETITION

1. Begin the Process with the Providers

The co-opetition effort can involve many diverse individuals and organizations, but the process should begin with providers. To make it work, they will, of necessity, be included, so it is best to start with a clear understanding that providers are at the core of the initiative. Breaking down historically competitive walls or getting over old grudges may be a bit challenging, but extending the olive branch of collaboration can have an amazingly disarming effect on even the most ardent opponent. At the outset, a driver or concept champion must bring the provider community together. If providers need documentation that the idea has merit, the article from *Health Forum Journal* on collaboration (Coddington et al. 2000) or a few copies of the book, *Co-Opetition* (Brandenburger and Nalebuff 1996), might prove useful.

Once the group has decided to meet, one individual should be designated to control the meeting, set the tone, and determine the agenda. To avoid territorial issues, this chief of the coalition can be either the one with most seniority in the field or the one with the longest tenure in the community.

The most important task of the founding members of the co-opetive covey is to first understand the rationale for and benefits from co-opetition. A clear understanding is needed by all the participants that the community will be better served and the players better off if co-opetition can become a reality. Although the initial projects or endeavors may be focused on one particular component of the delivery system, the group should understand that the end goal is to fundamentally alter the way healthcare is delivered.

The way the system has been set up involves so much inherent duplication and unnecessary inefficiency that providers need to correct the problem from within. The only way to permanently correct such dysfunction and fundamentally alter the delivery system is to come together on smaller initiatives and work toward marketwide standardization and optimization. Unfortunately, this industry is unlike the example of the technology industry mentioned earlier. In that instance, several major semiconductor manufacturers recognized the need for standardized practices and more user-friendly approaches and banded together to form Sematech. This was achieved from a financial as well as organizational standpoint because the size of the players and scope of the project facilitated its success.

That is not likely to happen soon on a national level in healthcare. However, it could realistically and readily occur among four or five market providers who recognize that, as the quote at the start of the chapter notes, "a rising tide lifts all boats." In this case, when competitors establish language, policies, standards, and evaluations that are more customer conducive, everybody benefits. That was essentially the goal of the Sematech initiative, and to some extent it worked. A similarly positive outcome can occur in healthcare once a shift in attitude and clarity of vision occurs.

If four or five providers are not able to make that mental shift toward collaboration or co-opetition, the process can begin with two or three. If the concept can be proven with fewer players, the opponents and skeptics may join when they can witness actual results from practical projects.

2. Identify Three Possible Co-opetive Initiatives

The next task is to identify three meaningful and achievable initiatives. This may take time, but it is extremely important. These three "opportunities" will be the group from which the larger coalition will choose, so they must all meet those two important criteria: meaningful—something that will have a significant impact on improving the community's health—and doable. Tremendous, untapped opportunities exist for co-opetive endeavors. As mentioned earlier, the first step is often collaboration. To that end, if organizations within the market are already collaborating on an initiative or two, that existing forum might prove the best avenue for organizing the coalition and initiating the co-opetition process.

The rationale for having only healthcare providers as the first players at the table is to provide a form of crowd control. The rationale for keeping the group "within the healthcare family" is to maintain control of the project and assess the feasibility of its completion before inviting collaborators that may not understand the complexity of the industry and the virtual impossibility of certain initiatives. It also enables hospitals and health systems to present the appearance of a united and organized front once the other members of the co-opetition coalition are invited.

In identifying the three alternatives, preliminary clarification of roles is needed. These roles should not be so much leadership roles (such as emperor of everything), but rather administrative roles such as communications coordinator (in charge of notifying others of meetings, taking minutes, etc.). The group should function like a community board, with projects selected that are achievable within a one- to three-year time frame.

The step of identifying three potential projects should take no more than a few meetings. If it takes much longer, the momentum will be lost and the concept will be challenged. The key component of these alternatives is to select projects that are meaningful and patently doable. As mentioned in chapter 2, to gain an early and relatively easy win right out of the gate is essential.

A good example of this might be to identify a mechanism for handling the swelling numbers of people seeking care in emergency rooms. This is a problem that has garnered considerable media attention in the past two years and is not likely to subside soon. Therefore, the initiative is one that is already quite visible, is viewed as a serious concern in many communities, and requires a collective effort to effectively implement.

Another possibility would be collaborating on a listing of doctors who are accepting patients. One health system in the Southwest developed such a list after soliciting feedback from area employers on what their employees really needed or wanted. The employers noted that although the area health plans provided listings of network physicians in documents beefier than a James Michener novel, the number of doctors actually accepting patients could not fill a pamphlet. This health system developed a separate list of only those doctors by working with other providers in the community, and the list was highly valued and much appreciated.

The above-mentioned endeavors are relatively noncontroversial yet could be perceived as significantly valuable, especially to the consumer. Ultimately, that is one important gauge of success for a collaborative or co-opetive venture—does it produce greater value for the community? If it does, nine times out of ten, the financial benefit will follow.

3. *Invite Nonproviders and Select the First Initiative*

Once the provider group has identified the three proposed initiatives, other members are invited to the co-opetive coalition. These new members would include complementors, including physician representatives, insurance carriers, employers, and perhaps government or local officials. Also included should be a few representatives of the customer segment—community members, employees, and patient advocates. The group is notified that they are part of very exciting and innovative initiatives to develop cooperative, market-based solutions to local healthcare problems. At the first meeting, the three proposed initiatives are presented, with the understanding that this represents only the first wave of possible solutions but that these are endeavors that the provider community feel are essential as well as achievable.

There are several reasons for broadening the group to include organizations outside the immediate provider confines. The first, and perhaps most important, is to realize the benefits of a communitywide consortium working toward a common goal or desired end. As the effort takes shape and the initiatives become more complex and systemic, a broad array of participants will be required to ensure the success of the project.

Another goal is awareness. The extent to which prominent people and opinion leaders within the community are involved in evaluating and reshaping the healthcare delivery system indicates the likelihood that it will reflect the needs and character of that community.

The broader group's role is to review the relevant issues and projected outcomes of each of the three initiatives and determine what resources each entity could marshal to successfully accomplish the task. Once the group has reviewed all three possibilities and made an objective evaluation, the group determines which of the three it will select. This can be done in a number of ways, depending on the makeup of the group and the culture of the region. One relatively simple and objective way is the Delphi method, in which individuals vote simultaneously but anonymously on the three proposals. The initiative with the most votes wins. Another way is to choose the initiative by consensus, but this may take more time. The time frame for winnowing down the selection should not take more than a few weeks. The preliminary group has already accomplished the hard work.

4. Develop a Resource List, Time Line,
and Accountability Matrix

The selection process is completed and the initiative is identified. The group is next charged with developing a resource
requirement list, time line estimates, and an individual accountability matrix. These documents are essential for evaluating the
progress and ensuring the successful completion of the cooperative initiative. These will also be widely distributed to the
organizations involved so that the individuals responsible will
be held accountable for their stewardship.

This is similar to most business planning processes, but once
again, the value of the larger group is the involvement with and
interaction among a broad spectrum of individuals and organizations throughout the community. These people are like sub-
committee board members for the initiative, and to the extent
that skills beyond or expertise outside the group are needed,
these well-placed individuals can tap into external resources.

Of the three components within this step, the most important
one from an accuracy standpoint is the time line. Establishing a
realistic time frame at this point, perhaps erring on the conservative side, is very important. If projects, especially consortium
or cooperative projects, go much beyond their expected completion date, the group becomes frustrated and the endeavor loses
some degree of credibility and cachet. It is better not to set the
time lines too ambitiously, as coming in ahead of schedule will
be a true mark of the group's ability to make things happen and
defy skeptics.

5. Secure Ample Publicity for the Initiative

The next step is to go public with the plan. The media is invited
to a coalition meeting at this point so that the scope and goals
of the initiative may be communicated. Meetings can also be

held with community opinion leaders to get the word out. This "broadcast phase" helps ensure two things. First, it holds the group's feet to the fire to get the job done, and second, it communicates to a wide audience that the community is working together to tackle a thorny issue of healthcare. This is a great opportunity for local healthcare providers to demonstrate that they are leading the charge in addressing the healthcare needs and issues facing their community. In so doing, they are extending themselves beyond their typically competitive boundaries and engaging many other key players in the dialogue, design, and deployment of solutions to relevant issues and individual concerns.

The entire arena of communication (discussed in chapter 5) is one in which many healthcare executives are neither comfortable nor adept. That is somewhat understandable, as the media has not always been kind to the hospital industry nor its leaders. However, as we embrace more tools for and encourage more forums on communication to our various stakeholders or audiences, we must become more skilled at conveying our message.

Nearly all members of the community will be receptive to this type of initiative. The public appreciates providers within the healthcare industry who are viewed as collaborators. In part, the concern over competition may reflect an intuitive sense (perhaps fueled at times by the media) that redundancy and waste in the manner of unnecessary duplication of necessary services is an inherent part of healthcare competition. For this reason and perhaps others, a press corps and public audience will likely be ready for and receptive to this kind of communication.

6. Complete the Initiative and Communicate the Victory

Once the work begins on the initiative, the larger group should continue to meet at predetermined checkpoints to evaluate progress, assess development, and adjust accordingly. This monitoring step, which is often overlooked and underestimated, is actually crucial to the eventual completion of the initiative. Progress evaluation will ensure that all the groups are not only engaged in the entire process but also well informed of the challenges in bringing the endeavor to fruition. It also serves to increase ownership and heighten appreciation for the effort involved in completing the project.

This very important phase occurs after the project is completed. A victory celebration should be held, with media invited and individual achievements acknowledged. This represents another good opportunity for the provider community to prove that collaboration is possible and—more important—beneficial. If the preceding steps are followed, this final step will represent the culmination of a well-known, highly regarded effort to not only bring the healthcare provider community together, but also to establish that healthcare is everybody's business—locally delivered and locally improved.

Healthcare needs to publicly celebrate more victories and recognize greater success. The industry also needs to be recognized for the great work already being done and the care now being delivered. Celebrations such as these allow healthcare leaders the opportunity not only to spotlight the collaborative spirit and the benefits derived therefrom, but also to highlight the day-to-day victories that rarely make the headlines but consistently enhance people's lives and improve the community.

The communitywide celebration also serves to elevate healthcare issues in the public's awareness. It provides an excellent forum for validating the maxim that all healthcare is local, both in terms of where to look for its delivery as well as its deliverance from the problematic issues and challenges the industry faces.

7. The Coalition Continues, Co-opetition Flourishes

The completion of the first initiative is just the beginning. The group continues to meet, as the concept must be embraced and engrained as fundamental to healthcare delivery. This is not a task force, but a perpetual coalition.

The temporary conclusion and celebration outlined in step 6 merely represents an opportunity to restart the process with one of the other two initiatives that were identified at the outset and continue the forward-thinking, upward-leading process to com-munitywide involvement and resolution of healthcare issues.

As the group moves beyond the earlier, easier endeavors, it can begin to tackle some truly thorny issues, such as reigning in the costs of healthcare, consideration of hospital districts or marketwide funding mechanisms, and even the mother of all problematic issues, dealing with the uninsured. This will be discussed in chapter 4. Suffice to say that one reason so many communities have struggled with these weightier and thornier challenges is that they have started out with projects that require very heavy lifting. The mind-set and mechanisms are not in place to galvanize and organize the collective to hoist in unison. Consequently, the parties become frustrated when they realize that even with their best efforts they cannot budge the bar off the ground.

Thus, the genius of co-opetition (especially in a provider-driven, locally based environment) is its facility to ease into the process with more readily managed issues. This allows the group to discipline itself, test its strength, know its weaknesses, and build its mass. It can then tackle the weighty matters that seem to be such a heavy burden on society but can best be lifted and leveraged at the local level.

APPLYING THE EXPERTISE OF OTHERS

The toughest thing is getting started, and the next toughest thing is maintaining the momentum. If organizations are struggling with trying to solve healthcare delivery problems on their own, they may want to consider forming a delegation to the "other sector." This would consist of organizing a coalition of a group of hospitals to embark on an in-depth study of operating practices at other industries such as technology. Examples of this kind of interindustry exchange already exist within our field (the automotive industry's involvement with healthcare in Michigan being just one), so the precedent has been established. You may think of it as a kind of "corporate foreign exchange" program. Realistically speaking, for many employers, healthcare is very foreign.

Another option is to invite a third-party facilitator or coordinator to get the initiative started and keep it moving. This will help eliminate any sense of favoritism and conflict of interest in the project identification. The third party could either be a local facilitator within the community or a healthcare expert who has extensive experience in collaboration. A few consulting firms and well-known individuals in our industry are available to offer innovative approaches to community solutions.

Whether the organizations choose to work through another industry, with a third-party coordinator, or simply on their own, the seven steps explored in this chapter can help them achieve a successful co-opetive effort.

SUMMARY OF THE STEPS TO ENHANCING THE SYSTEM THROUGH CO-OPETITION

- Begin the process with providers.
- Identify three possible co-opetive initiatives.
- Invite nonproviders and select the first initiative.
- Develop a resource list, time line, and accountability matrix.
- Secure ample publicity for the initiative.
- Complete the initiative and communicate the victory.
- The coalition continues, co-opetition flourishes.

EXAMPLES OF POTENTIAL PROJECTS

Of course, every market is different, but the following are some examples of co-opetive endeavors that are either being attempted in regions of the country or are under consideration:

- marketwide e-applications such as registration, scheduling, billing, and educational forums;
- agreement on data release, data sharing, or both to improve outcomes and increase public understanding;
- standardized physician credentialling for the entire market for all health plans;
- shared research and development expense to evaluate improved delivery models, increase access, and establish quality benchmarks;
- pooled resources to evaluate money-losing services (e.g., behavioral health) and offer single-facility or group-management options;
- standardized registration forms, admission procedure, billing options, and access protocol; and
- marketwide studies to develop more systematic, cost-efficient options to emergency room use, with follow-up based on educational efforts to redirect nonemergent cases.

How these goals are achieved is not nearly as important as the fact that they are achieved. The very act of forming this type of coalition to do something innovative and cooperative will be illuminating and productive. Furthermore, it sends a message to the corporate community that we as an industry are ready to listen, willing to adjust, and able to adapt.

In an industry known for its collaborative nature, co-opetition offers a viable option for retaining and upgrading the free-market model—healthy competition enhanced by a cooperative spirit and collaborative implementation.

NOTE

1. Portions of this chapter were previously published in the *Journal of Healthcare Management*.

REFERENCES

Brandenburger, A., and B. Nalebuff. 1996. *Co-Opetition*, p. 25. New York: Currency Doubleday.

Coddington, D., et al. 2000. "It Doesn't Come Easy," *Health Forum Journal* May/June: 34–37.

4

Increase the Number of
Insured to Enhance Income

*All that is gold does not glitter, and all that
wander are not lost.*

—J. R. R. Tolkien

IF EVER AN initiative called out "collaboration" or "co-opetition," it is one geared toward the uninsured. This serious problem has plagued the nation for years and within the past decade
has, in ebbs and flows, become the poster child for how broken
the healthcare system really is. It is the trump card that federalized medicine advocates (FedMeds) put out on the table when
they make their play for a nationalized health system. It is the
political equivalent of "remember the Alamo" come election
time or legislative session, and it is the one enduring dilemma
that probably receives more media ink than any other healthcare
issue.

However, when asked to list the top strategic opportunities
for revenue growth and income generation, few healthcare
executives would likely list "the uninsured." That may be a
matter of perspective or a question of semantics. Healthcare

75

executives do not get excited about the uninsured because they have a hard time envisioning how a group of mostly nonpaying individuals can do much for the economic betterment of their hospital. If any animation is evident, it is usually not very favorable, as they know that they are already taking care of this group increasingly every day through emergency room care. So while politicians, pundits, and patient advocates are theorizing and podium thumping, hospital executives are dealing with the problem by taking care of the population. As a result, when healthcare executives think of the uninsured, they may envision a nonpaying, fast rising, debt-loading population that politicians and statisticians have been haggling about for a decade but have not addressed.

ALTER THE THINKING TO FIRE THE IMAGINATION

This issue should be discussed as a matter of perspective and how we frame it. This chapter promotes increasing the number of insured, which is the same thing as decreasing the number of uninsured, but the messages these two phrases send are very different, and the potential interest in working with that group varies accordingly. The first statement merely conveys a diminishment of a serious financial drain, while the other represents the potential for increasing market share, expanding services, and better serving the needs of the community.

The topic of the uninsured is not as prominent now as during the months immediately preceding the 2000 presidential election, but it is still a thorny societal issue. Although the current dialogue is encouraging, the tardiness in spotlighting the topic is telling. Why has it taken so long to focus on the expanding number of uninsured and what could be termed a collective nonchalance in the body politic of American healthcare? Could the overriding obstacle be apathy? One recent participant at a major symposium in Texas on the funding of healthcare observed, "At least this year we're talking about the uninsured. At last year's symposium it wasn't even mentioned."

The lack of discussion may in fact lie at the heart of the issue, for the challenge of the uninsured is not new, even if it is now news. Recent Census Bureau findings confirm that their numbers have increased and the problem has intensified.

This chapter will present the case that this is an issue best and most likely to be addressed at the local level. At the national level, resolution is highly improbable. Anything short of nationalized medicine will be superficial window dressing, more geared toward the appearance of resolution than the accomplishment of it. The efforts thus far are commendable; however, the problem is so immense and the system so complex that finding a solution at the national level befits the classic description of a Herculean feat. The task is doable and the battle winnable at the regional or even state level, where most of the meaningful efforts are concentrated currently. This chapter outlines how a market or a region can address the concern and achieve the objective.

A VICIOUS CYCLE

Many people, even those within our own industry, do not realize we are in the throes of a vicious cycle, the consequences of which have debilitating ramifications for everyone. Much of the reason for this is the nature of healthcare in the United States, which is unlike any service or good in the nation because it is viewed as entitlement.

In 1946, President Harry Truman stated, "Healthcare should be a right, not a privilege." That sentiment has been perceptually adopted and legally supported. (Bill Bradley in his presidential campaign proclaimed that healthcare is "an American birthright.") Healthcare providers in this country are legally obligated to treat anyone who seeks care, regardless of the patient's ability to pay. The outgrowth of this right is that the costs for those who cannot pay are borne by those who can. Although such payment may be indirect and subtle, it is increasingly substantial. An example of this dynamic (and its ensuing financial consequences) is shown in Figure 4.1.

As depicted in this figure, the inherent and intensifying problem is that the current cycle of fewer insured is leading to increased ER visits. This results in substantial inefficiency in the system. An ER visit is far more costly to the overall system than the cost of a visit in a physician's office or an urgent care center. The dramatic difference in these cost calculations is shown in Figure 4.2. These numbers are extracted from data for Austin, Texas, but they are largely representative of most parts of the nation. Of interest, an estimated 50 percent of those treated in these emergency rooms could have been treated in a less acute and far less costly setting.

This inefficiency in the ER is but one example of how larger numbers of uninsured lead to higher overall healthcare costs. Who pays? Ultimately, everyone, but the first line of payment is borne by large corporations, the group that picks up the tab for the major share of commercial healthcare in the United States. One might ask, "Why haven't large corporations taken a more active role in shaping healthcare policy?" The problem has historically been the providers' to deal with, as employers have not linked the connection between the rising number of uninsured and the steadily increasing premiums. Yet, in a system in which the healthy and insured pay for those who are unhealthy and uninsured, a clear case must be made for a community solution.

ENGAGING EMPLOYERS IN THE DISCUSSION AND RESOLUTION

As mentioned earlier, one of the biggest challenges the industry faces is engaging the employer community. Any endeavor that

FIGURE 4.1: VICIOUS CYCLE

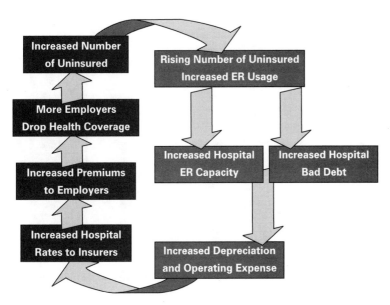

gets closer to achieving that formidable task is worthwhile. Increasing the number of insured may be one of the best forums for doing just that. Communities that have wrestled with this issue seem to have found a unifying focal point, a kind of galvanizing effort, from which providers can educate crucial audiences and marshal critical resources.

In the past, employers have distanced themselves from the healthcare dilemma rather than deal with it; they merely exhibit frustration and mounting concern. Few realize that it is in part their problem to own and not just their bill to pay. A communitywide coalition or task force organized specifically to address the seemingly impossible challenge of increasing the number of insured can be a source of illumination as well as a forum for resolution. Subsequently, it can enhance the financial picture for market providers and improve the overall health status of the community while reducing costs throughout the system.

FIGURE 4.2: COST COMPARISON OF GENERAL
MEDICINE VISIT

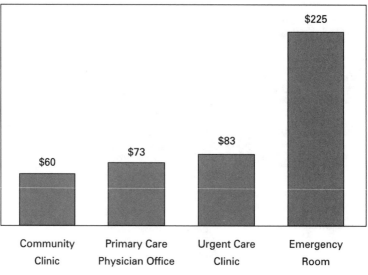

Source: Hospital Planning Department.

If representatives of corporations or even mid-sized businesses dedicated the same amount of resources to resolving
healthcare issues as they do with other areas of expense, they
doubtless would be more involved in finding and orchestrating
overall solutions. Just a few years ago the country was facing
double-digit increases every year in healthcare costs, as it is
now. One senior executive at a major corporation registered a
famous lamentation, "Our biggest threat to profitability is not
competitive innovation or strategy, but the rising cost of our
own employees' health benefits." That dramatic statement made
for a nice sound bite and an oft-referenced quote. However, it
produced little action.

In truth, if corporations in the United States spent one-tenth
the time and resources on healthcare costs that they do on product research and competitive response, we would see a dramat-

ically different healthcare landscape than we see today. This has recently been witnessed in the formation of the Leapfrog Group, a consortium of major employers dedicated to finding healthcare solutions. Arguably, no other entity could have a greater impact on the cost equation than corporations. That is why any suggested model or proposed solution that is likely to work over the long run must involve the employer-based insurance construct currently in place. Nearly 85 percent of uninsured Americans not of Medicare age receive their insurance through their employers. Consequently, any model that has a reasonable chance for success will pivot on the employer-based insurance system. Local, regional, and national models must have the participation of major corporations as well as medium- and small-sized firms in revisiting and refining the current healthcare delivery system and structure.

ENHANCE THE SYSTEM TO ACHIEVE INCREMENTAL SUCCESS

If the decade of the 1990s taught us anything about healthcare, it is that change must be gradual and progress incremental. The Clinton Health Plan proposal was too much for the public to swallow and the system to bear. Even officials within the Clinton administration admitted after the demise of the plan that their objectives were too ambitious and the required changes too dramatic. Interestingly, many of the underlying components of the Clinton plan have been instituted in the aftermath of its highly publicized defeat; they have been implemented on an incremental basis. Borrowing a cue from that experience, enacting a locally driven model that does not radically alter the existing landscape nor call for dramatic change is more likely to succeed.

To that end, two key elements currently in motion will likely be integral to the success of a regionally or locally based effort to handle the uninsured: local orchestration and incremental execution. As this book is being written, several states are developing or implementing programs that attempt to deal with this long-standing, rapidly swelling problem. Not all of these states are incorporating both these components into their model, but to one degree or another, a semblance of one or both can be found in most of the proposed models.

SEVEN STEPS TO INCREASING THE NUMBER
OF INSURED

1. Enlist and Engage Employers as the Driving Force

The first underlying element of a successful model for dealing with the uninsured finds its roots in a construct developed decades ago by some prominent patriarchs of the healthcare arena. The group first started meeting in the 1970s and was known as the Jackson Hole Group. Led by Dr. Paul Ellwood, a practicing physician in Minnesota known as the "father of HMOs," and Dr. Alain Enthoven, a Stanford economist, Jackson Hole espoused the notion of managed competition with a key component termed Health Insurance Purchasing Corporations or Cooperatives (HIPCs). The driving premise behind HIPCs was the pooling of employee lives to achieve greater leverage in managed care negotiations, heightened competition among health plans, and more efficient pricing through the spreading of actuarial risk.

Model the System After Group Purchasing Coalitions. A local coalition model or purchasing cooperative employs some of the same basic tenets of the Jackson Hole model, only without the federal oversight. In so doing, a local model can achieve the kind of efficiencies and economies that have been realized by purchasing coalitions. These range from the Buyers Health Care Action Group (BHCAG) in Minneapolis, which involves large employers, to the Coalition for Small Enterprise (COSE) in Cleveland, which includes more than 14,000 smaller firms. The latter has had an impressive track record of holding premium increases in the range of 3 percent to 5 percent per year while most small employers throughout the nation have experienced premium increases of 15 percent to 30 percent per year.

The cooperative or purchasing coalition can take many forms. As with the prior example, it can involve small- to mid-sized firms or larger firms. Or, as with one proposed model, it can begin with large firms that form a pool of employees and later add smaller firms once a sufficiently large pool is in place. In this type of model, the employer group that is most susceptible to untenable premium increase (small- and mid-sized employers) can achieve the same contracting clout or leverage as the larger firms, in essence, achieving parity in premium increases.

The other component of the uninsured model that is cropping up in many markets and several states involves a shift toward defined contribution. The concept of defined contribution, as opposed to the current model of defined benefit, is not entirely new to the American healthcare landscape, but it is starting to gain momentum. Defined contribution involves a model in which the employer contributes a defined amount of dollars toward the employees' health plan, but the employee selects the plan based on his or her needs. As employers grow increasingly frustrated with the challenges of administering health plans and angry at the prospect of absorbing double-digit premium increases, some executives of leading companies have expressed interest in getting out of the healthcare business entirely. The Xerox Company was one of the first to announce its intentions to switch to defined contribution in 1999. However, the firm faced such a backlash from unions and other groups that it had to backpedal on its original intention and revise its approach.

Defined Contribution and the Use of Vouchers. One of the major sticking points for employers opting for defined contribution is tax related. Under the current tax structure, the employer may not be able to claim an offset against revenue if it merely gives the employee the dollar equivalent of their current health benefit contribution. This is a significant hurdle for self-funded plans (which most large companies have) and arguably the biggest one employers face. However, efforts are under way to deal with this, and as interest mounts toward more creative and flexible solutions, even the tax issues and concerns will likely be overcome.

Defined contribution and a pooling of employees provide impetus for the concept of vouchers. Essentially, the voucher model (which has been incorporated by some entities, including BHCAG) allows employers to give their employees more interactions with the health plans they choose while reducing the involvement of the employer. This concerted effort to engage employees more in the decision-making process through the use of vouchers is theoretically and empirically beneficial to the system. The use of vouchers employs a model more like a traditional retail model, with greater accountability on the employees' part.

To make this work, the employers must be engaged in the engineering as well as the execution of the model so they can tailor it to the needs of their employees as well as the infrastructure of their organization.

Getting employers to the table is no easy task, given their track record of relative nonparticipation. However, if they can appreciate the potential cost savings in the long run for their organization, they will be more apt to commit time and talent to the process. To that end, local providers may want to develop their own graphs similar to Figure 4.1 to depict the costs of inefficient utilization and the impact such a disturbing trend as that shown in Figure 4.2 has on their organizational costs.

2. Establish a Purchasing Cooperative

The purchasing cooperative is fundamentally a community-driven, market-oriented approach to bringing more people into the ranks of the insured. The fundamental approach is to work though existing means of insurance and accepted channels of healthcare delivery. The goal is not to attempt a new model, but merely to tweak the existing one to make it more accessible and affordable to those who are not now able or willing to use it. One problem with many of the models proposed [such as medical savings accounts (MSAs) or tax modification models] is that they require too much change to the existing system.

As with HIPCs, the driving force behind the purchasing cooperative is a pool of employees of sufficient size to encourage managed care companies to offer competitive products. Large employers create the critical mass to form this purchasing pool by placing their employees in the purchasing coalition. Once the pool of participating employees is sufficiently large, small- and mid-sized employers can join the ranks of the insured. Thus, everyone is allowed access to reasonably and equitably priced insurance products, mitigating the current system of higher premiums for smaller employers, a result of actuarial-based risk adjustment. Consequently, employees of all participating firms are quoted premiums that are priced at a level previously reserved for larger employers.

Large employers are likely to come into the pool for two reasons: first, out of a sense of community benefit, essentially being part of the solution; second, and more realistically, because they recognize a need to be proactive in developing long-range solutions to escalating costs. By being a core part of the coalition, they are at the table, more actively involved, and much more engaged in the negotiating process.

The benefit for the small employers is obvious—they realize parity in the pricing of their health insurance premiums. This enables more employers to either offer or continue offering health insurance for their employees. Under this model, not only would smaller employers be able to receive competitive pricing, they would be in a better position to control premium increases rather than be subjected to the meteoric rises in health premiums they currently experience. Inherent in the cooperative model is also a tiered structure of benefits pricing that allows more companies to enroll at a more modestly priced cost structure and moves the market to more of a retail orientation.

3. Develop a Retail-Type Model Using Vouchers

As mentioned above, the other critical component of the purchasing cooperative is the attempt to shift healthcare to more of a retail model. This is accomplished through a voucher system. One of the most systematically troubling features of the American medical model is the financial and philosophical disconnect between user and provider. Much of this is caused by the reality that consumers (patients) do not pay full price for services rendered. Most Americans who have insurance pay a fraction of the total cost. Consequently, most consumers are not completely engaged in the medical decision-making process. The cooperative model attempts to repair this disconnect by encouraging more active involvement by employees and their dependents.

Under this type of model, each participating employee is presented with several options when purchasing healthcare benefits. These options are divided into four categories or levels:

platinum, gold, silver, and bronze. Each plan would involve a different benefit structure and an appropriate financial contribution. For example, the silver plan might involve a smaller deductible and lower copayment but would include fairly standard medical benefits. The cost of this plan would be in a range lower than that of plans currently offered by many employers. By contrast, the platinum plan would be higher priced than most models currently offered but would provide richer benefits, including alternative medicine modalities such as acupuncture and chiropractic. The cost would approximate that of the type of plan that executives in many companies now receive.

At the low end of the spectrum—and the level that would likely do the most to encourage smaller employers to participate—is the bronze plan. This would be a "limited benefit" offering involving a significantly reduced contribution by both employer and employee, with the total cost less than half that of the silver plan. However, the employee would only receive a very basic benefits package, such as primary care, catastrophic coverage, OB/GYN provision, and hospitalization or major medical coverage up to $5,000. Many of the enrollees in bronze plans would likely be individuals who are not currently insured at all. Therefore, this would be the area of greatest incremental gain in moving the uninsured into the ranks of the insured.

Importantly, one of the main objectives of enacting such a tiered model is to distance the employer from the decision-making process and enfranchise the employee. In so doing, employees should (theoretically) become more conscientious consumers, as they are in other services in which they have more of a financial stake. Insurance carriers would be responsible for developing products for all four categories and sell them individually to the employees through benefit fairs, e-mail transactions, or other means they may choose. Employees would choose from plans developed and promoted by three or four managed care companies, resulting in up to 16 different product choices.

Fundamentally, this type of model is designed to engage the engines of the free market, thus increasing competition and eventually stabilizing, if not decreasing, overall costs. This is why the voucher-type feature is vital to the model. Without it, any kind of employer-based initiative does not sufficiently alter the current out-of-sync model. This two-pronged approach is designed to utilize the existing framework to maximize the established network and to optimize the efficiency of a model that has been decades in the making. We do not need a new system; we just need to more efficiently use the one we have by increasing access, affordability, and accountability.

4. Involve a Wide Spectrum of Community Individuals and Enterprises

The committee or coalition that convenes to increase the number of insured should represent a broad spectrum of community interests and representative decision makers. To that end, a representative from local government, several representatives from the employer community, executives from the major healthcare providers, physicians, and adequate representation from the insurance community should actively participate. In addition, consumers should have a voice, either through individuals designated to represent their interests or by selecting someone prominent in the community who is outside the healthcare environment. The latter addition to the committee ensures that the language adopted, the message communicated, and the program developed will be understandable, consumer oriented, and tailored to the entity (i.e., consumers) that should drive the process.

By involving a diverse and representative group, the effort once again insures both greater buy in and increased understanding of the issues facing the healthcare industry. As noted in chapter 3 (and in subsequent chapters), these initiatives have dual benefit. They serve to inform as well as resolve. One thing the industry has learned from the Balanced Budget Act debacle is that the American public has little understanding of or appreciation for the issues facing healthcare managers today. Thus, a main side benefit of most of these strategies is education and communication (covered in greater depth in chapter 5).

The involvement of community leaders is an important precept and purpose to keep in mind, however, as providers are organizing and facilitating this coalition effort. Participants not only bring to the table resources but also the community clout they exert once they leave the room.

5. Assess the Current Situation, Tailor to the Needs of the Community

Once the coalition is sufficiently diverse and representative, the group should first assess the current state of affairs as it relates to the individual market. We often refer to this as an "environmental assessment." What are the key drivers in that particular community? Are small employers being forced to drop insurance coverage because of escalating premiums? Are health plans unwilling to offer products for small business or individual plans? These are questions that need to be answered in a fundamental environmental assessment.

The group may want to engage an outside party to coordinate the gathering of data and the collation of information. One of the larger health systems may have the internal resources (such as a planning department) to perform the task, but even if this is the case, it should not have to shoulder the entire burden. The advantage of having a third party involved is that, once again, it tends to remove the appearance of vested interest, territoriality, or skewed data. The costs associated with such an arrangement must be matched against the benefit derived.

Included in the assessment is information such as the estimated number of uninsured and how that number has grown over the past few years. Of course, the individuals behind the number are more important. Are these young people who are opting not to have insurance, or are they the "working poor," who simply cannot afford insurance or are not offered the option through their employer?

The environmental assessment process may seem to be an academic exercise, but it is actually essential. Too many well-meaning groups launch in a direction to change the course of their community without having a clear sense of the real issues or the drivers of the dilemma.

Critical to this process is market research or polling among the various groups affected by lack of insurance. This would include individuals who are currently uninsured or who have been uninsured in the recent past. Information to be gleaned from this group would include reasons for their lack of insurance, financial thresholds equated to the value of insurance, best means to communicate to these individuals, and general concerns and issues with the healthcare delivery system (such as access, language barriers, intimidation, etc.). Some of these may seem patently obvious, but an appallingly large number of these basic questions are not asked of the target population prior to launch of programs designed to meet their needs. This was demonstrated in a state where the launch of a children's health insurance program (CHIP) was promoted via electronic and print media. This proved both expensive and ineffective. Had the organizers of this effort surveyed those responsible for the notable successful Florida rollout of CHIP, they would have discovered that the most effective method of communication was grass roots—primarily through the schools. The state in question would have saved considerable money and likely enrolled considerably more participants.

6. Outline Solutions, Select, and Execute

Once this assessment is completed (and it does not need to be so thorough as to take months in gathering), the next step is to begin to explore possible solutions. Critical to this step is to review what has been tried before—locally as well as throughout the state and nation. Inherent in this process would be any statewide or regional initiative currently under development to address the issue. The community may need only to get on board with a statewide initiative to tackle the issue. If this is the case, the process is considerably easier and the required resources markedly fewer.

In developing proposed solutions, the group should consider bringing in experts from other regions or other states that have some experience in developing a similar model. This can provide valuable insight into the evaluative phase of the model. As mentioned with the CHIP program, the state in question could have easily consulted with the organizers of the Florida program yet maintained development of their own particular approach. There are no awards for creativity here. The goal is to succeed, and to that extent, learning from others' mistakes and good fortune will facilitate rapid execution and likelihood of success.

Once the group has developed three good options for approaching the dilemma, a discussion of the positive and negative aspects of each model as it applies to the individual community should take place. This is where the bulk of the time should be spent, as the selection process will largely determine the ultimate success of the chosen model. Too many groups rush this stage of the process and leap to a proposed solution, which is shortsighted and will likely prove ill fated. This is the stage at which the group gets fully engaged and assumes ownership of the proposed solution.

Once the group settles on one direction and one plan, the next step is to outline responsibilities and determine a time line for implementation. This phase is crucial, as it defines accountability and assigns ultimate responsibility. Nonetheless, this is a thorny issue and one not easily resolved, so the proposed time lines should be somewhat flexible. This is also where representation from local government comes into play, as it may require some legislative involvement from this critical constituency.

Through all phases of implementation, the important thing to remember is that the dilemma of the uninsured is a massive challenge and a complex issue. It is, therefore, highly unlikely that any solutions—whether local, regional, or statewide—will achieve significant success in the short run. The group should evaluate its success in incremental measures. For example, one goal of the group might reasonably be to stem the rising numbers of uninsured in the first or second year, which reduces the growth rate percentage. A more ambitious goal would be to actually increase the number of insured by a certain percentage over the first three years. However, to start out with an overly ambitious goal will only serve to frustrate the participants and derail the process. To keep providers engaged, the CFOs could estimate what impact the increased number of insured would have on their bottom line and on their overall financial performance. That number could be extrapolated for the entire market to determine how it translates to offering more services, improving the existing infrastructure, or (and this will be a tough one) holding down the costs for area employers. Those kinds of econometric models are becoming available, as more communities get some experience with these kinds of initiatives. A highly publicized venture is that taking place in Hillsboro, NC. This communitywide effort has garnered significant publicity and yielded impressive results by demonstrating that a community can come together and increase the number of insureds.

Other such models may be found throughout the nation, easily available by perusing the Internet and, for more in-depth study, by a personal visit.

7. Evaluate Incremental Results, Modify as Appropriate

The key to the overall effort is to recognize the important and inherent value of incremental success. One of the reasons so many of these initiatives fail is that the individuals involved want to solve the entire problem with one brilliant stroke, one blanket solution. Those do not exist—except in Hollywood scripts and politicians' platforms. Finding a universal remedy to this dilemma is like trying to drain a lake with one cup. Progress will be slow, so organizers should expect modest results and should celebrate minor victories. They will be less likely to become frenzied and frustrated and give up when the process seems to be moving too slowly and accomplishing too little.

Also important to this phase is constant evaluation of the endeavor as it proceeds. Again, organizers should not be opportunistic, lest they radically modify the game plan before it can be effectively executed.

The final phase of continually evaluating incremental success and modifying the model while adjusting the process is almost as important as the early design phase. As new programs are developed that emerge from the federal and state government, the local model must coincide with those initiatives and augment existing or planned programs.

SUMMARY OF THE STEPS TO INCREASING
THE NUMBER OF INSURED

- Enlist and engage employers as the driving force.
- Establish a purchasing cooperative.
- Develop a retail-type model using vouchers.

- Involve a wide spectrum of community-based individuals and enterprises.
- Assess the current situation, tailor to the needs of the community.
- Outline solutions, select, and execute.
- Evaluate incremental results, modify as appropriate.

Some might reasonably ask, "Why should providers lead the charge on this issue?" That statement is both telling and confirming. It is telling in that it demonstrates that we are not known for, nor used to, coming to the table with communitywide solutions. We must alter that way of thinking and that mode of operating. It is confirming in that it should be the very thing we spend our time and our resources on—community solutions to health-related problems. If nothing else, even the exercise of gathering a representative group together to explore the issue of dealing with the uninsured will send a crucial message to community leaders that providers are willing to commit intellectual and financial capital to developing overarching solutions to underlying dilemmas.

This chapter essentially promotes three reasons to undertake this initiative. First, it is the right thing to do, and no one sector or entity can orchestrate a solution better than the provider community. Second, it sends a powerful message to the community that providers are about more than just money. Third, if the problem is not addressed soon, the financial fallout will be severe. The rapidly rising number of uninsured individuals will likely capsize many hospitals and health systems and could eventually sink the private-market healthcare system in the United States.

5

Use Communication as an Economic Tool[1]

*What we have here is a failure to commu-
nicate.*

—"Cool Hand Luke"

IN MOST CONTEXTS, communication may not be viewed as
a strategy, especially not an economic tool. If anything, it is
more likely to be viewed as a mechanism or a means to execute
other strategies. However, in healthcare, we have for the most
part done such a poor job of communicating that the activity
of communication itself needs to be viewed as a strategy. The
goal is to elevate its significance and its pivotal position in the
strategic portfolio.

Some within the industry may bristle at the earlier statement
that "we have done such a poor job of communicating." In
truth, that may be overly complimentary. Ask a neighbor or an
associate who does not work in this industry to explain what
makes healthcare work and why it does not seem to be working
well right now. A recent article in *The Wall Street Journal* discussing the Institute of Medicine study was entitled "Healthcare

Services Are Inadequate." (Lueck 2001). The harsh reality is that most people in the United States have no earthly idea what our healthcare system is all about—or what we are doing to improve it. This is not meant to demean our expertise or diminish the role but to give a candid assessment of a disturbing reality. This reality must serve as a backdrop against which we can measure our current strategy and future commitment.

SEVERE CHALLENGES ARGUE FOR BETTER COMMUNICATION

There has never been a more important time for us to marshal our individual and collective resources in an effort to communicate more openly, frequently, and effectively. Heathcare executives are facing more situations that require tough choices and, therefore, better communication. One example comes to mind: A well-known and highly regarded health system in the Southwest recently refused to sign a Medicaid managed care contract. The negotiated rates of the contract were well below the cost to provide the services. However, many of the enrollees in the Medicaid plan still used the services of this particular system, largely through the ER. When the health system billed the managed care company for out-of-network services, it received a "reasonable and customary" rate that was actually unreasonable and incendiary—reimbursing about 15 cents on the dollar. So the question became, should the system sign the contract, recognizing that rates are well below cost? Or should it in effect draw a line in the sand and refuse to sign, all the while realizing it will provide services to the same individuals at unattractively low reimbursement rates?

Although this anecdote may be more dramatic than most, this type of scenario occurs in markets throughout the country on a weekly basis. In addition, with the federal government increasing its involvement and intervention and managed care players trying to recoup sizeable losses, we are likely to see many more tough-call situations. How should hospitals and health systems respond? The traditional response has included the tried and perhaps not-so-true methods of legal action, government advocacy, and good old-fashioned indecision.

In terms of legal action, the health system mentioned above is taking the managed care company to court, suing for a more reasonable rate. The problem with this path is twofold. First, the process is lengthy, distracting, exhausting, and usually inconclusive. Second, the courts have demonstrated a reticence to get involved in healthcare business matters.

An even more common method for redress is to seek political intervention and legislative action. This course, while sometimes productive at the state and perhaps even national level, is ponderous by design, global in nature, and more frustrating than assembling kids' bikes on Christmas Day.

Some executives attempt to address such seemingly impossible situations by delaying communication or by parsing out just enough information to ward off the media or to "not say anything that could get you in trouble." Such an approach stems from the mistaken notion that if the situation is so difficult that no feasible solution presents itself, the system should wait until one does. In essence, "delay the inevitable by foregoing the unpalatable." Although industry executives may be hesitant to admit it, the minimal communication/delayed action method may actually be the most commonly practiced response to tough-call situations.

A SOUND LESSON FROM A WISE MAN

However, none of these methods produces meaningful results in a reasonable time frame. Given that, perhaps we need to look to the embodiment of good decisions in tough situations, King Solomon.

Unfortunately, we do not have too many King Solomon–type case studies to review, but what we do have is instructive. Most people are familiar with the Bible story in which Solomon was asked to judge between two women, both claiming to be the mother of the same infant. Because the king was wise but not psychic, he decided he needed more data to make the decision; thus he proposed the impractical (and gruesome) solution of dividing the baby in half. The imposter responded with a cavalier, "No problem." The real mother, however—her protective instincts overriding her custodial interests—yelled out, "No! She can have the child." At that point, savvy Solomon, having concluded his focus group study, turned the baby over to the legitimate mom.

This instructive story actually has considerable implications for the several situations that require tough choices and extensive communication. Fundamentally, Solomon's solution was all about communicating consequences to the affected parties. To make the call, he needed more input from the individuals who stood to gain or lose from his decision. He needed to make them aware of the consequences of the outcomes.

A similar dynamic must occur in healthcare, and the fact that we have been remiss to undertake such a process probably has many people outside the industry wondering why.

THE APPLICATION TO HEALTHCARE

When we read about a hospital or health system that is sustaining serious losses, filing for bankruptcy relief, or just shutting down outright, one cannot help but wonder if the executives in charge were communicating their situation throughout the ordeal. Admittedly, some problems land hard or move fast, but many troublesome situations develop with ample warning and sufficient lead time.

The problem with last-minute solutions to long-brewing crises is that they tend to produce reactive responses that are by their very nature dramatic, expensive, and stopgap. In such cases, the affected parties, who end up dealing with the situation, resolving the crisis, or experiencing disruption, have a legitimate right to question why it ever got to the point of emergency. This oft-repeated situation is reminiscent of an adolescent who, on Wednesday night, informs his parents that he has a term project due on Thursday morning. Oh, and by the way, could the parents provide some much-needed, late-night assistance?

In the case of the procrastinating adolescent, we can all relate to the folly of youth. However, a seasoned executive charged with the stewardship of a community's health coming to responsible stakeholder groups at the eleventh hour with a serious crisis is another matter altogether. Individuals and organizations have a right to question judgment and challenge reasoning. As the managerial maxim goes, "Try never to let someone else's poor planning become your emergency." Yet for many community leaders and public servants (board members, city officials, and so forth) it does become their emergency and they have a right to wonder how it escalated (or deteriorated) to that level.

It all boils down to communication. For the most part, we have not done a very good job communicating the changing state of healthcare and its effect on our individual facilities. We have been reluctant to pull back the curtain and allow stakeholders to *see things as they really are* and how changes could affect their lives and their community. By not communicating more openly, we may have done our community a disservice, and in the process, we no doubt have retained an enormous burden.

THE MEDIA AS A VEHICLE, NOT A PARIAH

Many of our problems actually result from a "failure-to-communicate syndrome." An important step in successfully shifting from a culture that offers minimal, reactive, or no communication to one that uses communication as an effective tool is attitude realignment toward the media. Observation of this industry indicates that more than a few hospitals and health systems maintain a belief that the media intentionally reports negative stories about them. Therefore, media representatives and contacts are seen as something to be avoided at all costs. The following anecdote from a multihospital system is symbolic, if not representative.

The system hired a new communications vice president. Within a week of his arrival at the system headquarters, he received a phone message from his assistant notifying him of a call from a newspaper reporter. The assistant said, "Do you want to just ignore it or should I tell her you're not available for a comment today?" When this newest member of the management team looked somewhat stunned by her approach, the assistant said, "Well that is how we usually deal with the media."

The communications vice president soon learned that in this particular case, one of the system's board members had been burned by the media—or at least he felt he had. Consequently, paranoia and sometimes outright animosity toward the media spread throughout the entire organization to the point that media calls were usually avoided and *never, ever,* initiated.

This situation is not an anomaly, and although it may not be the norm, it is far more prevalent than it needs to be. The problem with the "under-siege-by-the-media" mentality is that it often spills over into other communication venues and with other audiences. Hospitals and health systems do not have to open their organizational curtain wide and reveal everything to be seen. However, the historically held and often-practiced approach of steering clear of the media, thus failing to communicate with critical audiences, is detrimental and poor strategy.

This industry is viewed as complex and largely closed to outside scrutiny. Such an industry, especially in an era of information and communication, is fundamentally incongruent with the vast majority of American enterprise. This incongruity may be one reason why a strong push is being made by various groups to "pull back the curtains" and provide more information on everything from outcomes data to pricing information. Based on current trends, we are likely to either open the door for greater examination or be forced to open the door to inspection.

RELEASE OF DATA AS OPPORTUNITY OR THREAT

Indicative of this is the push for the public release of data, which has already occurred in some states and is forthcoming in many more. This sweeping movement, feared and loathed by many healthcare executives, seems unstoppable. Of course, the Internet, with its unprecedented ability to facilitate communication readily and universally has also broken down many barriers with such vehicles as online report cards and detailed information on providers. Now, physicians are fighting to keep their comparative data from the watchful eyes of anyone who has access to a computer. The struggle is probably useless, as in time such information will inevitably be available.

For years, healthcare executives and physicians have argued that the release of such data is "dangerous in the wrong hands and before the wrong eyes." The rationale is that healthcare is so complex that the data reporting mechanisms are somewhat spurious and that the lay public is not capable of objectively interpreting the data. That the industry has been able to fend off publishing the data with such a circuitous argument for as many years as it has is amazing. However, time and reason have caught up with us.

The same argument could be made for the airline industry, or, for that matter, just about any industry that can make a reasonable case that the average person cannot interpret comparative data. That may explain why nearly every other industry in the United States has made the comparison of its services simple, understandable, and capable of communicating at a rather rudimentary level. What we in healthcare do not acknowledge is that opening the data door has the potential to become a great blessing for this industry. It will force many more organizations to communicate, evaluate, and operate in a fashion that can be understood by the outside world. At that point, the differences between providers can be communicated to the average American — without the necessity of wading through something as complex as JCAHO tomes or HEDIS data, or taking the time to get a degree in medicine.

SEVEN STEPS TO USING COMMUNICATION
AS AN ECONOMIC TOOL

*1. Adopt an Attitude that Communication
Is Central to Strategy*

The first step in transitioning an organization from one that has historically built up communication fortresses to keep relevant and useful information inside is to recognize that the same organization now wants to build portals to broadcast relevant information to the outside. That requires a definite shift in attitude, approach, and operational style. The question becomes not so much one of *whether* to communicate as *what* to communicate, and *when*.

To make this shift, the senior executives should "become converted" to this principle by understanding and appreciating the benefits of open communication. If the payoff is not apparent, the initiative will garner few true believers. The truth is, the payoff for open, frequent, and effective communication is real and sizable. The public wants to know more about what happens in healthcare settings. They are more than willing to be forgiving about the favorable or unfavorable nature of the data and not so willing to forgive lack of accessibility of the data. In other words, healthcare managers have assumed that withholding data is better than risking presenting data that places the organization in an unfavorable light. The latter, incidentally, is a misconception. As the old saying goes, when nothing is communicated, one usually assumes the worst.

One way to make the transition easier and more pervasive is to understand and communicate the economic value of frequent and effective communication. A concerted communication plan will not only prevent some very expensive situations but also, if done effectively, can be the means by which the organization attracts incremental customers in its existing markets. It can also be the catalyst for expanding into new markets, such as complementary medicine, and increasing the number of insured. The reason for pointing this out in the first step is to establish up front that gaining complete buy-in to a communication plan as central to the strategy belief may lie in quantifying the value of such a strategy. In essence, this determines in bottom-line significance the impact of a sound and solid communication plan.

2. Appoint a Communication Czar or Chief Communications Officer

Another way to get the senior staff buy-in and organizational support is to designate a chief communications officer (cco) or communications czar. The communications officer can be the marketing vice president, a public relations director, or someone particularly gifted at and interested in the communications function. The role of the cco is to coordinate the overarching communications initiative as well as to shoulder ultimate responsibility and accountability for its successful completion. Most organizations already have someone in this role, or one akin to it, but that role may not be elevated to the necessary status required to effect a communications turnaround within the enterprise and as it relates to the outside world.

Make the CCO *Part of the Executive Team.* The CCO should be a part of the executive team within the hospital or health system. Anything less than that level of organizational status will likely result in a communications rollout that is less than optimal. The CCO needs to be aware of and involved in the main directives and key initiatives of the organization. He or she must not only be a communicator of those initiatives but a key contributor in the development of them. Communication needs to be a theme, not an afterthought, of an organization that is committed to recognizing its economic value. Of course, this can be taken to extremes: a leading not-for-profit system based much of its strategy on how it would appear in the public light. The system made some fundamental errors because what played out well from a communications standpoint did not work out well from an economic or operational execution standpoint. For example, the system in question jumped the gun more than once by announcing an initiative in the press and later backpedaling on the announcement for lack of effective execution. It should be noted that this represents an extreme that is rare in this industry. Typically, communication is given the short shrift.

The key is to find a balance. Much of American enterprise is marketing oriented. From service industries to manufacturing, communication—in the form of promotion or public relations—is always a leading consideration before any initiative is launched. Too often in healthcare, it becomes a matter of consideration *after* the decision to initiate a change is made and the service is configured, not while the evaluation and development are underway. A highly placed and well-respected CCO can help ensure that communication is an integral part of the analysis, as well as the execution of expanded services, revised programs, or new initiatives.

3. *Conduct a Communications Audit*

Once the CCO has been designated and appropriately placed within the organization, the next step is to conduct a communications audit. This important component can be completed by surveying members of key audiences or stakeholder groups. This would include representatives from employer groups, insurance companies, physician groups, government organizations, and the community. The survey could also include vendors, public health officials, politicians, and essentially any group the organization thinks is vital to its ongoing success.

One caution in this regard is to limit the number of stakeholder groups to four or five. Otherwise, the surveying or marketing can take on a life of its own and result in a never-ending process with a seemingly bottomless pool of prospective respondents. Importantly, a small sample size can represent those stakeholder groups that are surveyed. Being pragmatic is important when considering market research: conducting a reasonably representative survey—brief, inexpensive, and directed—is more important than a "statistically significant" survey that can prove expensive, overly exhaustive, and academic.

Survey results will form the backdrop against which the communications plan is developed. Without the benchmarks provided by such a study, knowing what messages need to be emphasized as well as how to determine and measure the ultimate effectiveness of the communication effort is practically impossible.

The number of organizations that do not periodically survey their key audiences or stakeholder groups is surprising and disconcerting. Although many hospitals and health systems regularly conduct attitude and awarness surveys for their market among the public, other audiences are too often ignored or forgotten. How many health systems have polled employers in their area to find out how they feel about the services offered in the community? How may hospitals have queried managed care organizations to determine how they regard the delivery component of healthcare in their area and what matters most to them from a quality standpoint? The answer is that very few poll these critical audiences. Therefore, they have little idea as to how they are perceived by these groups.

So it is with the four or five key audiences the organization identifies in this step. The survey process does not need to be extensive or exact—especially at the outset. It just needs to get done. Once accomplished, the cco and his or her colleagues will have baseline information on which to assess the market and gauge their success.

4. Develop an Organizationwide Communications Business Plan

The next important step in the process is to develop a communications business plan. The communications plan should be well understood and thoroughly distributed among members of senior and middle management. The development of the plan alone will elevate the relevance of communication as a key initiative in the organization's strategic portfolio. As with any plan, tactics should be defined in quantifiable terms, with accountability matrices and time line parameters.

As part of development and drafting of the plan, the organization should consider appointing a committee with broad representation. As with previous strategies that involve multifunction groups, the committee's diversity should help ensure not only a broader perspective but also greater awareness and acceptance. The communications committee or work group assigned to oversee and execute the plan should meet periodically to assess the progress of the plan and to adjust accordingly.

In addition, organizations should consider an advisory group with representatives from within the organization as well as members of stakeholder groups to provide valuable feedback on clarifying insight into the process. Representatives from outside the organizations provide two valuable contributions. They offer additional perspective, and they serve as a constant checkpoint to ensure timeliness of completion and appropriateness of effort.

5. Execute the Plan with a Type of Medium Appropriate to Diverse Audiences

In the past, too many healthcare executives have maintained that communication to the outside world is the sole purview and prerogative of the marketing or public relations department. Consequently, the communications strategy was often confined to a printed brochure or a well-placed billboard. An effective communications plan entails much more than that.

Many ways are available to get the word out and the message across. One likely forum is, of course, the media. Many healthcare professionals and organizations are media-averse. Such shyness, which for some is outright paranoia, may be understandable, but it is largely unproductive, especially now when the public demands more forthrightness. In most markets, the media is not only highly interested in healthcare happenings, it will likely be objective, reasonably understanding, and professionally intrigued. Local situations may differ, but the healthcare sector is usually one of the top five employers in most areas, so interest is inherent. Importantly, communications initiatives cannot be relegated to national press and industry associations. If we truly believe that healthcare is a local phenomenon, our communications effort must be locally based and community specific.

Other important and instructive forums are available for communicating our message and educating key audiences. Many communities already have some forum for employer roundtables. Such forums may involve CEOs or human resources directors. Whatever the audience, the forum is a good medium for communicating change in an interactive way, allowing healthcare leaders to spend as much time listening as informing. Employers are still paying the tab for most privately financed healthcare, so they have both a financial interest and a community concern. Unfortunately, the number of healthcare systems or hospitals that regularly meet with employer groups is disappointingly low.

Other avenues for this type of invaluable communication include educational mailers, hospital-based programs, and Web-enabled information. Community chat sessions offer real-time discussions with real people for audience feedback and innovative suggestions. The form and forum are not as important as the concept of open communication. By indirectly admitting that, like Solomon, we may not have all the answers, and by candidly offering a peek inside our world, we broaden the decision-making base and alert people to the consequences of probable outcomes. All these audiences, along with the appropriate messages, can be a part of an overall strategy and a comprehensive communications plan. Affected parties can then be galvanized into action, much as the real mother who manifested her maternal instincts and turned Solomon's tough call into an easy decision.

6. Evaluate the Success of the Communications Initiative and Adjust Accordingly

A critical part of the program's success will consist of a post-execution evaluation and correction. This should be conducted to determine the effectiveness of the plan as well as provide direction for the initiative going forward. The communications plan should be a dynamic document, describing a never-ending, constantly upgrading process. There is no final completion date, but only interim evaluation stages. Consequently, this phase of the planning process involves a cycle of assessing, adjusting, adapting, and beginning the endeavor all over again. This is one area that is too often the victim of minimal energy and nominal time. Yet organizations that truly capitalize on their communication strategy take this step very seriously—perhaps more than the others—and derive great benefit from doing so.

7. *Quantify the Economic Impact and Celebrate the Incremental Gains*

One of the reasons healthcare organizations seem to experience stutter-starts with their communication initiatives, whether through marketing, education, or public relations, is the failure to quantify the benefit. Therefore, when times get tough and money gets tight, the communications component is downsized or dropped altogether. The reason this does not happen in other industries (where marketing is often the last thing to get cut) is that they understand the long-range danger of such a short-term reaction.

Taking their cue, then, from other industries, healthcare executives would be wise to assess the financial impact and potential of communication strategies. Some would say that such measures cannot be obtained, but that is almost always untrue. Even if the analysis consists of something as basic as the incremental value of one additional point of market share, such measures can be estimated, if not calculated fairly accurately.

Additionally, there is the all-important calculation of what a good communications plan saves, or what lost opportunities result from a poor or nonexistent strategy. What revenues and profits are lost when the sponsoring organization fails to effectively communicate to hold market share or fend off competitors? For example, one large system decided that an extensive marketing campaign to ward off a newly arrived niche player was not worth the expense (or, more aptly stated, investment). The loss of revenue and profit—both directly from that particular service line (cardiology) and from the spin-off business—proved exponentially greater than the cost of the campaign would have been.

Such calculations and considerations are routine in other organizations yet rarely determined in the healthcare industry. The economic term "opportunity cost" is the difference between the financial benefit from the current strategy and that of an alternative strategy. Healthcare executives would be prudent to factor in the notion of opportunity costs, as well as potential gains, when evaluating the quantitative component of communications strategies.

SUMMARY OF THE STEPS TO USING
COMMUNICATION AS AN ECONOMIC TOOL

- Adopt an attitude that communication is central to strategy.
- Appoint a communications czar or chief communications officer.
- Conduct a communications audit.
- Develop an organizationwide communications business plan.
- Execute the plan with a type of medium appropriate to diverse audiences.
- Evaluate the success of the communications initiative and adjust accordingly.
- Quantify the economic impact and celebrate the incremental gains.

Of the many items on the industry's to-do list, open and candid communication should be near the top. If done professionally, succinctly, and successfully, such an effort can rally the allies, buttress the organizational bulwark, and stave off market and regulatory forces that present challenging choices.

Most industries outside of healthcare realize that they are basically reduced to nothing if they cannot effectively communicate. For some it is their reason for being. As an industry not very adept in this particular area, we would be wise to once again learn a lesson from our corporate colleagues in other sectors. Healthcare leaders may better recognize that effective communication is the underlying foundation on which sound operational strategies are built, revenues enhanced, and profitability increased.

NOTE

1. Portions of this chapter were published previously in the *Journal of Healthcare Management*.

REFERENCES

Lueck, S. 2001. "Healthcare Services Are Inadequate." *Wall Street Journal*, March 2.

6

Derive Financial Benefit from Complementary and Alternative Medicine

Greater than the force of armies is an idea whose time has come.

—Victor Hugo

WHEN HOSPITALS AND health systems started to seriously consider offering complementary and alternative medicine (CAM) about four or five years ago, little excitement for the concept was noticed. If anything, considerable concern, if not resistance, was evident. Now, the issue for many hospitals is not *whether* to offer CAM, but *how* to provide the services in a way that is politically astute and economically sound.

THE COMPELLING ECONOMICS OF CAM

For those who may not have noticed CAM's increasing presence as a potential strategy, providing a little background and a few reasons for considering the concept may be helpful. The first and foremost rationale for developing some kind of CAM presence is economic. Research conducted by David Eisenberg of

Harvard estimates that CAM expenditures account for around $25 to $30 billion dollars (Eisenberg et al. 1993). Those familiar with the CAM movement will remember that Eisenberg first pegged the economic value of CAM. His study, conducted in 1991, placed that value at approximately $14 billion. Of that, approximately 75 percent were out-of-pocket expenditures, comparable to the total out-of-pocket expenditures for all physician visits in the United States during that same period.

When Eisenberg and colleagues repeated the study a few years later, he found that the number had swelled to nearly twice that of the original estimate and was on pace to continue growing at a much faster rate than conventional medicine (Eisenberg et al. 1998). This is an especially interesting statistic in light of the fact that most of the expenditures are not reimbursed, so no "multiplier" factor exists. In other words, the growth of CAM is even more impressive because people are willing to pay retail for it. That element alone should communicate why healthcare executives need to consider embracing alternative medicine.

OTHER IMPORTANT CONSIDERATIONS

There are other reasons why hospitals and health systems need to consider CAM as part of their strategic portfolio. Obviously, consumers are highly interested in the services, as they are clearly voting for them with their pocketbooks. Yet the group of consumers utilizing the services is particularly interesting. Although CAM usage cuts across all demographic sectors, the largest concentration is among baby boomers. Boomers have changed the face of every other industry in the United States and emblazoned their inimitable signature on the way these companies do business. They represent a demographic group that is both massive in size and atypical in character. If the boomers are embracing CAM, healthcare executives would be wise to regard such a significant migration from conventional medicine, as this could very well be the signature statement the boomers place on traditional healthcare.

RESEARCH VALIDATES STAYING POWER
AND GROWTH POTENTIAL

Another reason for considering incorporating CAM, which aligns with the boomer phenomenon, is that CAM is not likely to diminish in popularity and economic significance in the near future. It is not a fad that will pass in time, like the current fascination with televised survivalist shows and instant millionaires. Extensive research was conducted in the late 1990s among both "light users" and "heavier users" of CAM that produced some very interesting findings and served to validate its consideration (St. David's 1997). Light users were defined as those who had either just recently started exploring CAM modalities or had only used one form of CAM treatment. Heavy users constituted the group that had been purchasing CAM services or products over many years or multiple modalities. Even among the latter group, however, little cross-utilization among CAM participants was found. For example, those who used acupuncture were not necessarily prone to utilizing other modalities, such as herbs or chiropractic.

Another important finding of the focus group research was that among the participants of CAM, the major barrier to incremental (i.e., more frequent) use was economic, not interest or desire. In marketing parlance, the demand was not saturated, as participants had not yet arrived to the point of multiple modality use, nor was their demand satisfied by availability on single-modality use. This means that the market for such modalities has a great deal of growth potential among its current users, not to mention those who have not yet tried CAM.

BROADENING THE PORTFOLIO OF SERVICES

The final reason to incorporate CAM into strategic planning and implementation is the benefit of bringing on new services to expand the portfolio. By incorporating CAM in some form, the organization is forced to design its operational architecture to different specifications. This exercise is both instructive and essential. Implementing CAM provides a good test model for the organization to gauge how readily it can adopt new services and adapt to shifting market tastes and trends. This is foreign territory for many healthcare executives, but it is an important venture to consider. CAM represents a good vehicle for testing the waters because it is just different enough to make the organization stretch, but not so far outside of the traditional milieu that it requires an entirely different set of skills and a new configuration of the delivery system. Although CAM does require minor modification, it does not require a radical reconfiguration.

Therefore, CAM represents an opportunity for an experimental launch. As long as organizations do not go to market with an overly ambitious effort, the endeavor should be complementary, just as the name indicates. As with most facets of healthcare delivery (and as mentioned several times throughout this book), an incremental implementation is best, with minimal modification and moderate promotion.

NOMENCLATURE AND MODALITIES

Defining a few rudimentary precepts and parameters of the CAM movement and market considerations may be helpful at this point in the discussion. One of the first questions to surface is, "What is the appropriate name for these services or modalities?" That is a relevant question, as some sensitivity to the nomenclature does exist. Several names for this field could apply. A partial list of names by which the area is called include the following: unconventional, holistic, natural, Eastern, new age, integrated, and, of course, complementary, and alternative.

Exactly where the term CAM originated is a question for debate. Arguably, it has become the most popular reference for the field. One explanation based more on observation than on actual definition is that physicians and conventional practitioners bristle at the term "alternative." Even those in the medical community who accept or even advocate CAM modalities (such as Dr. Eisenberg) do not like the term, as it implies that they are a substitute for traditional medicine. Furthermore, practitioners in the actual field of CAM do not particularly like the moniker alternative because the word carries other associations in current society.

Consequently, both physicians and CAM practitioners, such as acupuncturists and herbalists, tend to prefer (at least in the past few years) the term "complementary." However, the field has long been known as alternative, dating back decades, so far less name recognition is shown with "complementary" than with "alternative." As such, the combination of complementary and alternative is a somewhat practical compromise to assuage the professionals and connect with the public. The term has been given credence and exposure by its use in trade publications and leading conferences. The aforementioned Dr. David Eisenberg hosts an annual conference at Harvard on the subject. That conference serves as both a beacon and a bellwether for the field, as it has the cachet of Harvard Medical School and the practical confluence of many practicing CAM professionals. His group started using the term (although they may not have originated it) in the late 1990s, and it seems to have taken root. Additionally, the focus group market research mentioned previously surveyed people on their preference of names (St. David's 1997). The responses from the CAM users validated the assumption that most people refer to the modalities as either alternative or complementary, so the combination pretty much covers the waterfront.

One further consideration has come to the fore: some physicians bristle at calling this field "medicine." Healthcare executives may encounter that kind of resistance, depending on their particular market. Admittedly, this type of resistance is less prevalent than it was several years ago, but more traditional markets may find it a sticky issue. One way to counter the concern is to note that whether it qualifies as medicine is very likely a moot issue. The public refers to the services as "alternative medicine" or "complementary medicine." Resistant physicians will not change the public's opinion nor the field's nomenclature. If resistance to the naming of the endeavor is still detected, it may be helpful to prove the point with local research (discussed later in this chapter).

CAM COMPONENTS OR MODALITIES

The next major question often asked is, "What exactly qualifies as a CAM component or modality?" Perhaps no one can definitively answer this question, as it is largely subjective. However, for healthcare executives the question is fundamentally academic, as at the present time only a handful of modalities should be considered by acute care organizations.

CAM can be divided into modalities that range from "established" (e.g., chiropractic) to "nonthreatening" (e.g., massage therapy) to "politically radioactive" (e.g., crystals). This kind of delineation may help the sponsoring organization sort out the modalities. The established modalities would be those that have been around for a long time and are quite prevalent in American society. Chiropractic is the best example of this, as it has the largest following and the highest awareness. Yet chiropractic is somewhat controversial among some members of the medical profession in some areas of the nation. Some physicians see it as competition, others as ineffective. True skeptics—those who come out of their chair at the mention of its name—consider it quackery.

Nonthreatening or politically innocuous modalities are those that do not stir as much emotion among physicians, nor as much potential controversy among traditionalist board members or staff. These modalities are not viewed as competitively threatening, but rather as therapeutically complementary at best and physically innocuous at worst. This classification is exemplified by professional massage therapy. Not many doctors bristle at the work of professionally trained and expertly qualified masseuses. Acupuncture can also fit into this category in many areas, as it has become more widely accepted—even practiced—among physicians.

The politically radioactive therapies are those that could be viewed as on the fringe of medical practice. These therapies might range from the mystic to the questionable. One writer in the field termed these "Berkleyesque." These modalities may have merit or sizeable followings; however, aligning them under the umbrella of the medical model is not worth the risk. When discussing possible services and products within the CAM portfolio, these services are best left off the table.

The timing regarding the introduction of these various modalities is another consideration. Some are appropriate to offer in the first stage of development and promotion, while others should be introduced in the second or third phase. Those modalities considered politically radioactive can be eliminated immediately.

What *is* relevant to consider in modality selection is that five of the modalities, according to research by Dr. David Eisenberg (1993), account for over 80 percent of the total expenditures in the field. These heavy hitters, in terms of volume and revenue, are as follows:

1. chiropractic (by far the big revenue producer);
2. herbal medicine (the fastest growing modality);
3. massage therapy;
4. acupuncture; and
5. self-help or self-care.

Other CAM modalities may be offered along with, or as an adjunct to, these more prominent components; however, these five represent the anchors for the CAM mall, so to speak.

EFFICACY LIES IN CUSTOMER EXPERIENCE

One of the issues that will sometimes come up is the lack of scientific evidence that these modalities actually work or that they are efficacious. This issue is highlighted by an anecdote involving a young graduate student who was serving an administrative fellowship for a Florida hospital CEO. This young man called a recognized expert in the field to discuss a project. He told the experienced executive that his system was considering a CAM initiative and his assignment was to gather sufficient clinical research to prove the efficacy of the techniques. The CAM expert told him not to waste his time searching for clinical data for two reasons: First, he would not find much (although more evidence may be available now). Second, and more importantly, it was really a moot issue because consumers do not require such data, as indicated by the fact that over one-third of the population is using CAM modalities without it. The veteran told him that if he was trying to get the data to assuage the doctors or to justify offering CAM services, he—or the hospital leadership— was heading down the wrong path, and the other competitors in the market would leave them behind.

The lesson from that story is to not wait for clinical proof of efficacy to begin developing CAM initiatives. The public does not want it, and regulatory agencies (at least for now) are not requiring it. The rapid growth of CAM is proof enough that something is working. Furthermore, the field has achieved this success with relatively little advertising and very little organization. Admittedly a fair amount of promotion for herbs and supplements has been seen. And, indeed, chiropractors have been promoting themselves for decades. For the most part, however, CAM practitioners are even more balkanized and fragmented than traditional or conventional medical practitioners are. Consequently, very little organized or centralized promotion or education has taken place in the last decade. The growth in this area has come largely through word of mouth.

This last reality came to light in the focus group research when survey participants were asked how they found out about the modalities they were using. Nearly all of the respondents commented that they heard about their particular modality from someone they knew and who "swore by its effectiveness." Few, if any, had heard about the modality from advertising or more broad-based means of promotion or education.

THE PHYSICIAN'S SIGNIFICANT ROLE IN CAM

Any organization considering CAM initiatives is strongly urged to work toward ensuring physician awareness. At the same time, sponsoring hospitals or health systems should not be delayed by a few doctors who expect or demand to see clinical proof that CAM techniques work. The reality, based on people's experiences, is that they do work.

Furthermore, as Dr. Eisenberg—one of its chief advocates among the medical professions—stated in a speech on CAM at the Harvard Symposium in February 1997, medical doctors need to have discussions about the use of CAM with their patients. Even if physicians do not believe in the efficacy of the modalities, their patients are very likely accessing CAM services. Dr. Eisenberg maintains that physicians must discuss the use of

such modalities with their patients so they can more appropriately coordinate their overall care

Consequently, Dr. Eisenberg's main message to physicians is
that, even if they do not believe in the concept, they need to
speak openly—not patronizingly or critically—to their patients
about what CAM practitioners are doing and how that care may
blend with the care the doctor is recommending.

Interestingly, focus group research conducted by St. David's
(1997) substantiated and corroborated Dr. Eisenberg's sentiments and approach. When the respondents were asked how
open they were with their personal physicians about their use of
CAM, most replied that they did not discuss it with their doctors.
They felt that their physicians would not accept their use of
such practices. However, the vast majority of the research group
commented that they would have liked to discuss it with their
personal physician, provided the doctors were supportive of such
behavior.

LARGE BUT DIFFICULT MARKET

For all the seeming attractiveness of CAM—fast growing, fragmented, cash business—the harsh reality is that it is a tough
market in which to flourish. One of many reasons for this is the
political risk. As mentioned earlier, many physicians bristle at
the very thought of CAM modalities associated with the hospital
or health system. This is no small issue. Some healthcare executives have chosen to ignore the very important consideration of
physician resistance and have subsequently launched a major
CAM initiative at their peril. One thing should be well understood at the outset: In the short run, CAM represents a relatively
small revenue stream. There is no reasonable rationale to risk
the economics of the health system on what some would term
"pocket change." Stated another way, it is not worth betting the
farm on a crop of small potatoes.

A few executives have taken that gamble, and lost. A policy-maker may say, "But this book declared that it was such a great strategy." It is a *good* strategy in the short run, if done with the right level of stakeholder awareness, acceptance of ownership, and incremental execution. In the long run, and for the benefit derived from attempting the effort, it is a *great* strategy and one that merits serious consideration.

SEVEN STEPS TO DERIVING FINANCIAL BENEFIT FROM CAM

1. *Form a* CAM *Committee to Evaluate the Options*

This may start to sound like a broken record, but the first step is to form a committee or task force to review the feasibility of CAM. If the group determines it is worth pursuing, it can develop a business plan for the initiative. This group should consist of at least one senior executive who can take recommendations and progress reports to the executive committee of the hospital or health system. A few clinicians should be involved as well as a marketing and financial representative to assess market readiness and economic viability, respectively.

A broad cross section of hospital employees is once again relevant in terms of the need to access resources as well as ensure awareness and commitment. The greater the representation (within reason, so that the group remains manageable), the greater the likelihood of support and eventual success.

The CAM committee has two important functions. One is to act as the investigative force behind the initiative. This group determines the viability of the endeavor and challenges assumptions. However, once that is done, the group needs to be its strongest advocate and champion. Therefore, assembling a group that is analytical and objective, but not resistant or intransigent, is important. Otherwise, when the time comes to take the concept to the execution phase, the rest of the organization will pick up on the hesitancy or outright resistance to CAM. This caution comes from empirical experience: One health system thought it was doing the right thing by inviting an outspoken critic of CAM on the evaluation team. The naysayer played an important role during the analytical phase but was never able to make the transition to concept champion and eventually undermined the overall effort with his negativism.

2. Obtain Physician Input and Support

One of the first things the CAM group should do is test the water with several groups. One such group is obviously the physicians. This is probably best accomplished in small groups that, if possible, include medical doctors who will champion one of the less controversial modalities. This might be a doctor who believes in or practices one of the modalities. In one market, a health system found a psychiatrist who practiced acupuncture. This doctor was well respected for his medical practice, so acupuncture, which usually is not as politically dangerous as, say, chiropractic, was viewed as acceptable.

Another option is to involve doctors, such as sports medicine specialists or general orthopedists, who routinely refer patients to massage therapists. Of all the modalities, massage therapy is the least likely to raise concerns among physicians. Typically very few physicians have a problem with licensed massage therapists, but even this view should be tested on a market-by-market basis.

Once an M.D. champion, advocate, or practitioner is found (and this individual might even serve on the CAM committee), he or she should serve as the key communicator with the doctors. Experience teaches that M.D.s are much less prone to immediately criticize one of their own—at least openly—and more likely to at least give them an audience. Yet they will still be candid with one of their own, just not quite as caustic or vitriolic as they might be with a healthcare executive or clinical manager who is advocating the initiative

3. Conduct Market Research Among the Public

Once the physicians have been surveyed and informed, the next group to poll is the public. This can be done through focus group research or quantitative surveys (e.g., phone surveys). Holding at least two or three focus groups is recommended. These smaller groups serve several purposes. First, the sessions will very likely be illuminating for senior executives and members of the medical staff. Ideally, the initial focus group respondents should consist of users of CAM modalities.

As mentioned in the section dealing with early market research conducted in this area, it is a good idea to have one or two groups with more frequent CAM participants or multiple modality users, and one or two with light users—either recent "converts" to CAM or single-modality-use individuals. The latter group will provide some insight into the growth possibilities of the market as well as insight into how they found out about CAM.

If possible, it is also interesting (but not necessary) to interview people who have yet to utilize a CAM modality. This group of nonusers will provide insight into the barriers for these people, as well as possible strategies on how the health system may eventually tap this incremental market.

In conducting the research, several important aspects of the endeavor can be determined. One of the most important deals with physical setting or location. For example, the focus group participants can be queried on their interest in and affinity for having CAM providers located close to or affiliated with existing healthcare organizations. The research by St. David's (1997), cited earlier, produced the clear finding that CAM participants did *not* want such modalities offered in traditional medical settings. This finding was not only revelatory but highly relevant, as the sponsoring health system had gone into the research hoping to offer the CAM services and modalities in their urgent care settings.

In this case and for this market, the focus group participants stated quite emphatically that they thought such a setting was too "sterile" and far too "clinical" for CAM modalities. That should have been fairly obvious, but it turned out to be somewhat of an epiphany.

Another important variable to test is the desire to have multiple modalities offered under the same roof or in close proximity. Again, one might intuitively believe that such a setting would be desirable, but the research by St. David's revealed that some modalities were far more complementary and geographically compatible than others. One important principle to learn from this early market research is not to assume anything and not to develop the design of the system or the model on intuition.

4. Evaluate Existing Networks

Once the market research is conducted, the next step is to survey the market for existing practitioners. An existing preferred provider organization (PPO) may consist of CAM practitioners. If so, this offers an opportunity to either align with such a group or present a competitive option. CAM providers—whether organized or not—may be looking for an opportunity to gain more clout or obtain a centralized location for their services.

A few years ago, CAM networks, whether in PPOs or other configurations, were relatively few. Now they are springing up in major markets across the country, as practitioners recognize the value of economies of scale—both for promotion purposes and contracting clout. Consequently, tapping into one of these existing networks could prove instructional and may save a great deal of time on the organizational front.

That a network is simply in place does not provide reason enough to align with the group. Considerations for partnership or merger should include reputation of the group, contract arrangements, legal ramifications, and potential for synergy. For example, if the market already has a network of CAM providers, the fundamental question is, what added value does a partnership with the health system or hospital bring to the community, the practitioners, and the system itself? If there is no economic differentiation (such as contract negotiating clout), no increased public exposure (via the marketing expertise or resources of the health system), and no upgrade in overall status of the CAM network, the affiliation may not be in all parties' best interest.

5. Develop a Plan for Implementation

The next step following the development of a network is to create a phased-in plan for offering the services. Again, the operative word is incremental or gradual. Some systems have chosen to start with something as politically innocuous as educational classes to ease into a CAM program. For many markets, this would probably be too conservative, as the public and physicians involved are beyond showing great concern over the idea of a health system sponsoring CAM services. Between the heightened awareness of modalities (primarily over the past five years) and the efforts of physician advocates like Dr. Eisenberg, doctors seem to be more tolerant than just a few years ago. Nonetheless, "easy does it" is a good theme for this initiative, and sticking to the more accepted, less controversial methods of CAM is far preferable to creating an organizational maelstrom.

In addition to the organizational and marketing components of the plan, the CAM effort should have a solid financial plan, but not one that is expected to bring in vast hordes of customers nor to make monumental profits. It should be viewed more like a start-up company—an investment in the future that will take some time to achieve a reasonable level of profitability.

6. Consider Hiring External Management

CAM represents a new way of delivering, promoting, and operating services. Although it is medically related, it is a different venue from traditional medicine. The environment is different, as is the expectation. For example, research revealed that CAM participants expected a softer, less "scientific" or sterile setting. They expect to spend more time with the practitioners. That expectation indicates one reason so many people (according to focus group research conducted by St. David's 1997) are turning to CAM. They like the personalization and face time that is perceived as declining in conventional medicine.

Given that, as well as the divergent nature and personalities of CAM practitioners relative to medical doctors, the sponsoring hospital or health system might want to seriously consider finding someone outside its organization to launch this enterprise. Candidly speaking—and again based on empirical evidence from other nontraditional initiatives—many healthcare executives are too conservative, too engrained, and too limited in their vision to effectively run such an operation. That is not meant as a criticism as much as a direct observation of what the industry has experienced either in the CAM realm or other areas like physician management organizations.

An organization may indeed have the internal management strength to handle such an assignment. However, the organization should give prolonged and extensive consideration to that first manager—and not assume that the individual has to come from inside the ranks. Some existing personnel can transition easily, but those staff members are often found in the middle manager ranks—not necessarily in senior management, where the assignment is often placed.

7. Continue Support, Build the Program

Once the effort is implemented, making sure it receives sufficient support—in terms of both attention and promotion—is highly important. Many of these initiatives get launched and rolled out to the market with great fanfare but with insufficient backing. After six months of disappointing performance, senior executives look down on the venture and say, "See, we told you it would never work." They become the victims of self-fulfilling prophecy and self-inflicted provincialism.

Maintaining the momentum and keeping up the support throughout the entire implementation phase is also very important. This can be accomplished best by incorporating a scheduled plan for staggered offerings, coupled with a willingness to keep the initiative going even if the results after the first few months are not as promising as expected or desired. A staggered introduction makes good business sense, as it tends to lower the expectations and concentrate the effort, and it gives all the more reason for a three- to five-year plan, rather than just a reactionary jump-start.

As the effort takes shape, gains volume, and approaches profitability, some of the earlier steps can be repeated, especially market research among existing and prospective consumers. Dialogue can also be pursued with managed care companies to consider offering CAM modalities as part of the local health plan. Managed care support is once again starting to build. Such support and backing began to take shape a few years ago when Oxford, Kaiser, Wellpoint, and a few other major players announced their intention to bring CAM modalities into their plan portfolio. However, when managed care experienced its financial setbacks in the latter years of the 1990s, CAM exploration and inclusion were some of the first efforts to get the ax. Now that some of the larger managed care companies are posting more favorable financial results, a renewed interest in and support for including CAM in their plan is surfacing. Even if insurance carriers do not modify their traditional plan offerings and reimburse for CAM, the market for such services seems only destined to grow at a rapid clip. The baby boom generation is approaching the age span where the body breaks down at a seemingly geometric pace. This will place a strain on the capacity of the entire healthcare system in the United States, and because CAM seems to be one of the signature health items for boomers, the outlook for this field is quite promising. It is likely to continue to grow at a more rapid rate than conventional medicine and therefore should be on the to-do list of every far-thinking healthcare executive in the United States.

SUMMARY OF THE STEPS TO DERIVING FINANCIAL BENEFIT FROM CAM

- Form a CAM committee to evaluate options.
- Obtain physician input and support.
- Conduct market research among the public.
- Evaluate existing networks.
- Develop a plan for implementation.
- Consider hiring external management.
- Continue support, build the program.

As with many of the previous initiatives discussed in this book, part of the value of CAM is found in exploring the concept and embracing a new kind of regimen. Here the management is the message. And the message is that the hospital or health system is willing to change with the times, adapt to the market, and conform to customer interests and specifications. That is an important message to send in these times of rising consumerism and declining favorable perception in the healthcare industry. A CAM initiative will probably not radically alter perceptions or financial performance, but it is a very important step in a long journey that needs to be started very soon. Additionally, it falls within the mission of most healthcare organizations to improve the health status of the community. As more Americans look to CAM for improving or maintaining their health, it is highly important that the leading institutions in the nation are part of that movement.

REFERENCES

Eisenberg, D., et al. 1993. "Unconventional Medicine in the United States." *New England Journal of Medicine* 328: 246–52.

Eisenberg, D. M., et al. 1998. "Trends in Alternative Medicine Use in the United States." *Journal of the American Medical Association* 280 (18): 1569–75.

St. David's HealthCare Partnership. 1997. Focus Group Research Study. Austin, TX: St. David's HealthCare Partnership.

7

Take Economic Advantage of Retail and Visual Traffic

If fate does not adjust itself to you, adjust yourself to fate.

—Persian proverb

THE CONCEPT AND application of retail and visual traffic is one of the driving forces behind many of the technology juggernauts, entertainment concerns, and prosperous industries throughout the world. Nonetheless, it still is primarily vanguard strategy for most healthcare organizations and will therefore not be taken too seriously by many tenured executives. This concept is one of visual traffic, presence, or "image."

We live in a marketing- and advertising-oriented world. Many people do not know the difference between the two; suffice to say that marketing and advertising are *not* synonymous. Marketing is much broader and significantly more strategic than advertising, yet many in our industry still fail to recognize the difference, so this chapter will make references to both.

Advertising and marketing have fundamentally driven the entertainment industry to its unparalleled prosperity. Additionally, they are part of the driving force behind the unprecedented popularity of athletics—collegiate and professional.

THE EYES HAVE IT AND THE DOLLARS SHOW IT

If you do not believe that the popularity of athletics is relevant to the concept of visual traffic, you probably have not attended an athletic event lately. The visibility of the Olympics, any major sporting event, or the entertainment taking place during the Super Bowl is all related to commercials. The event, the athletes, and the competitive contest are largely a backdrop for the real show: the sponsors' opportunity to entertain, impress, and persuade. This is the source of funding and the fuel that fans the flames of promotion.

Taken on a broader scale beyond athletics, marketing may be the single biggest driver behind the long-running prosperity of the nation. Consider the major firms, the dollars they spend, and the influence they have on the world's spending habits, especially those of Americans. Think what would happen to this country's economic engine without the ubiquitous marketing presence of McDonalds, Coca-Cola, Disney/ABC, General Motors, or Microsoft. World leaders come and go, but worldwide marketing companies are everlasting, or seemingly so. Furthermore, if an organization can somehow get one or more of these types of marketing-driven behemoths interested in what they are doing, they can tap the marketing wave that washes over the world.

Nearly every industry in the United States other than healthcare has come to understand the economic reality that visual traffic accounts for modern-day wealth generation. That is how Amazon.com—without any foreseeable profit and not much revenue—captured Wall Street's fancy, *Time's* "Man of the Year," and the abject sorrow of investors who speculated that the innovative start-up could become an established blue chip. In the aftermath of the dot-com meltdown, pundits may well ask, "What were we thinking?" The answer is quite simple: Here is a new medium for transaction, and just as important, a medium for consumer traffic, or "eyes."

The same could be said for athletic contests, entertainment showcases, or any event that attracts a large viewing audience that can be influenced to spend sizeable amounts of money. It could not be said, however, in healthcare.

Healthcare managers and executives appear to be remiss or reluctant to embrace this principle, not to mention the opportunity. Consequently, we once again remain on the fringes — unable or unwilling to capitalize on a movement (call it a phenomenon) that has captured the attention of consumers and the creative application of marketing executives throughout American enterprise. Too many of us fail to grasp the significance of traffic, hits, or images.

ISN'T HEALTHCARE DIFFERENT?

Why the healthcare industry for the most part has not grasped the concept of leveraging the vast number of people who walk through their doors, visit their patients, and see their facilities is not clear. Some might be thinking, "But we do — we have a gift shop." Although that may be helpful, it is comparable to a football stadium with little more than hot dog booths, program vendors, and parking attendants. The money at those games is not made merely by selling a little food, a few programs, and a parking spot a little closer to the game. The money, as athletic organizations throughout the country and enterprising companies throughout the world have learned, is made by selling the audience a series of messages, a variety of sundries, and, lest we forget, the event itself.

The first thing to do in considering this strategy is to think about how other industries and enterprises use their position and leverage their presence to maximize value to their audiences. Some might be thinking, "Yes, but we're different. We don't want to do that kind of thing." The fact is that some hospitals and health systems already are, and more will follow.

Hospital Organization and Management

We live in the information age, where the central consideration is communication. Yet as an industry we have not tapped into the wealth of opportunity available nor transformed our organizations in a way consistent with most of American enterprise and with worldwide trends. As we begin the process, we will not only provide economic benefit to our hospitals and health systems, we may just stave off the forces that are calling for federalized medicine, an option that is not only suboptimal but against the drift of other developed nations.

SEVEN STEPS TO TAKING ECONOMIC ADVANTAGE OF RETAIL AND VISUAL TRAFFIC

1. Assign Organizational Accountability for Retail and Visual Traffic

How do we capitalize on a trend that is integral in nearly every other industry in the United States? The first step is to appoint or hire a true image expert. This can be a marketing or advertising specialist or someone who has experience in another industry where visual traffic is a staple and a source of significant revenue. This expert may be found in either the business development side of the technology sector or in the promotional side of retail. Filling the slot with someone within the organization will probably be difficult, as it truly requires a different mindset and an array of separate skill sets than are usually found in healthcare senior management.

The image expert must have a definite retail style, which is sometimes an anomaly within the industry, as it requires a much more commercially focused orientation. Although the prospect may seem daunting, such people can be found. A good candidate may have run a restaurant or worked for a national chain of stores. Yet finding those types of leaders in middle and senior management is not as prevalent in healthcare as it might be in other industries. This individual needs to have astute marketing *and* advertising skills, as well as retail acumen.

Fundamentally, this individual is charged with leveraging the amount of traffic — pedestrian as well as visual — that traverses the organization on a daily, weekly, monthly, and yearly basis. The first task of the image expert is to calculate the number of people who come through your facility or facilities on a periodic basis. One relatively modestly sized hospital in Missouri calculated the number of patients, visitors, family members, and others passing through its hospital at approximately one-half million a year. For a city of less than 100,000 residents, that number surprised even the CEO, who had estimated the number at a fraction of that.

Physical traffic in most healthcare facilities alone is impressive. Getting a good quantitative sense of the immensity of the figure will provide a retail specialist with a fairly good sense of what he or she can expect to do with the services to be offered. As will be discussed below, the number will likely be broken down by service line or department, but the aggregate is a good place to start.

The next important calculation is that of other types of traffic. This would include people who frequent programs sponsored by the organization or attend classes or educational seminars presented by the health system. These may be offered off campus or in satellite facilities. This will likely be a number far lower than that representing those who actually walk through the facility or facilities, but not an insignificant one.

Visual traffic includes people who see the facility or its affiliated clinics, offices, programs, or delivery vehicles. In addition to actually seeing the physical surroundings, thousands of people in the community will see various promotional pieces or literature. And of course, the web site, if the hospital or health system has one up and running, provides another view.

When all the numbers are calculated, the final figure is aggregated to present to potential "partners" that would benefit from and compensate for having their messages in front of the millions of eyes that will see the organization's image and relate to its position in the community.

2. Assemble a Team or Committee on the Retail Initiative

Once the visual traffic/retail czar is found, he or she should assemble a team of individuals who can assist in developing the business plan for retail and visual traffic. This endeavor can eventually be viewed as a service line with an attitude—or at least a different approach. The group should include at least one senior administrator and a broad cross section of organizational representation, including finance, marketing, clinical expertise, and—very important—legal or risk management counsel. The legal issues will become particularly important for most organizations as the group may develop ideas that challenge tax status or mission fit.

The team's task is to follow the same type of regimen and preliminary evaluation that has been described in previous chapters. This would include listing possible options and arraying them in some form. A portfolio grid could serve as a graphic representation of these options, using axes such as ease of entry, potential profitability, capital requirement, political sensitivity, synergy with other service lines, and compatibility with organization mission. Depending on which measurement criteria matter most, the grid could depict each option using these metrics. Perhaps two or three grids, listing different criteria for the axes, could be drawn up and a percentage weight assigned to the relevance of each grid.

However the initial assessment is done is not as important as the fact that it gets done. The value of listing several options in this area and arraying them in a semiobjective fashion is immense. Otherwise, often the "idea of the moment," the latest front-page story on *Modern Healthcare,* or the pet project of a doctor or senior executive is chosen as the project to launch. The problems with that approach are obvious, but the bigger danger is that, should the inaugural venture fail, the entire concept will be scrapped, tainted by the first failure—all a result of a subjective selection process.

3. Test the Concept Among Many Audiences

Once the grids have identified one or two strong candidates, market research should be conducted. As with other initiatives, the research helps corroborate the committee's intuition as well as identify major stumbling blocks or political land mines. For that reason, testing not only prospective customers but other audiences that might be affected by these ventures is important. For example, in the case of a retail unit, the sponsoring organization would definitely want to survey the doctors. They may view the endeavor as anything from unprofessional to competitive, depending on the nature of the venture and the conditions in the market.

Keeping other stakeholders apprised, if not involved, is also important. One of these audiences is the board. It may seem rather obvious that the administrative staff would inform its board, even solicit its input prior to progressing, but some have either chosen not to or simply did not think it important. A highly disgruntled board member can kill a reasonably good idea much faster than poor financial performance. It is best to keep them informed and ensure they are aware of and comfortable with the plans.

Other audiences that might merit consideration in the input and informational phase would include employers (they also might see the venture as competitive or demeaning), managed care organizations, and, of course, the regulatory and legal agencies or organizations.

4. Launch with a Program Involving Low Commitment, High Probability of Success

Every market is different, but starting off with some sort of retail component that is relatively nonthreatening and requires a low resource commitment is probably the best bet. Several hospitals and health systems have begun this effort already and can be consulted for their experience and observations. One hospital in the Southwest set up a retail display/sales unit in its maternity ward, where it distributed items for nursing mothers and paraphernalia for newborns. This unit has performed much better than expected, netting over $60,000 in its second year. This is doubly impressive considering its low-key approach and no-pressure sales orientation. Little additional effort is involved by the staff; the nurses provide some technical assistance in explaining the products and services.

The success of this particular unit is worth noting for two reasons, both of which make a strong argument for the concept itself. This particular unit has done well because it meets a need at a critical time for the customer. It is the perfect example of being in the right place at the right time. Additionally, the retail setup within the confines of the maternity area allows mothers and others involved in the newborn experience to access the expertise of true professionals, not minimum wage clerks who may or may not know much about these products. Given that the audience for these products may be new to this experience and the necessities that go along with it, the value of expert advice makes this milieu the perfect setting for such a setup.

Many such examples can be found across the nation, and an entirely new offshoot industry is springing up to tap this market. As mentioned, it is one in which the patients (in the case above, new moms) know relatively little and have access to experts (i.e., nursing staff) who know much and are available for the advice. That same logic applies to a number of service areas and product offerings.

Start Small, Build Gradually. As with other such services, the administrative staff should adhere to a business plan that provides a three- to five-year time frame in which the initiative has a chance to bear fruit. Much like the CAM initiative, the retail component should start out small. If the group launches with a mammoth effort that involves a great deal of publicity and disruption, physicians and even some patients are likely to loudly object and accuse the hospital of too much commercialization or even profiteering.

The response to that type of criticism (even if it comes from a somewhat subdued or minimalist effort) is that this is what the patients want. That statement is not fabricated; that is what the aforementioned hospital in the Southwest found out through its market research. If the sponsoring organization wants to verify that finding, it should conduct its own market research or can initiate the process based on the findings from other markets.

The hospital or health system must exercise caution in just how far to take this concept. A lesson can be learned from the fast-moving, high-flying Columbia/HCA. In the mid-1990s, that company started developing retail health centers in malls, with a focus on health-related women's products and paraphernalia. The company launched a site in Florida with hopes of taking the concept to a national level. However, the pilot site failed. In the aftermath, the managers admitted that although the idea was sound, the location was flawed and the rapid execution premature. As with so many new ideas, it is far better to start small and build than to begin large and crumble.

5. Look for Partnerships for Visual Traffic

Once the retail component is sufficiently under way, the image czar and his covey of creative colleagues can focus their attention on leveraging the volume of traffic that patronizes the health system or hospital. This can be done in a number of ways. One way is to solicit those who might be interested in visual images, namely, advertising sponsors.

Advertising sponsorship is admittedly new to healthcare, so the bugs have not been completely worked out, nor have all the political land mines been completely defused. Nonetheless, local organizations should have a sense as to what will work and what will not. For example, some hospitals have entered into joint ventures in which they use their good name and solid reputation as image capital for the venture. Just by loaning their name, they avoid having to put up monetary capital to the venture or can invest at a reduced level.

In the past couple of years, it has become vogue for major corporations to "lend" their name—and a great deal of money— to hospital wings or components of a hospital, like the children's hospital or the women's pavilion. Another venture being explored in Texas and other parts of the country is the concept of a "health village." Although admittedly still in embryonic form, the architect of the idea has obtained financial commitments from some fairly strong players to develop a kind of ambulatory medical mall. The village would feature many of the services and amenities one would find on a large medical center campus, only in a more urban and relaxed setting. Like a medical version of a Barnes and Noble, it has much more ambience, with all the resources one could hope for.

One of the premises of the health village is that advertisers are willing to pay a premium for signage and for presence. The concept is still to be proven, but the idea has merit and the precedent is certainly established for other industries and services. Based on the experiences of other health systems and the sponsorships of major corporations, the concept appears to be taking root.

Some hospitals are recognizing the value of signage on their hospitals. Again, some farsighted organizations have been doing this for years, but placing large banners or tastefully developed and designed signs or marquees on prominent external locations is a great way to maximize favorable location and leverage many visitors. As an industry we are poised to take the concept to another level and allow other complementary businesses and services to tap into the signage issue. A few years ago, no one would have thought much of this concept, but with the Internet leading the way, it is worth looking into.

6. Use the Internet as a Prototype

As hospitals consider leveraging their presence in the community and affording corporations or other sponsors the opportunity to benefit from it, they should look to the Web as a model. For example, the web site for HCA, eHC, is planning to leverage its significant presence in millions of homes by commercially offering space on the site for local services and national concerns. There are likely other applications for this concept in other mediums that have not been tested yet or are still in the development phase for vanguard healthcare executives. Achieving what other industries and myriad organizations have been doing for years—namely, providing their audiences with more (and relevant) information for a fee—simply takes some creative thinking and application. In marketing parlance, this is called virtual cross-selling: the customer is exposed to complementary services that are offered by a different company but still have application to the core service being provided.

Of course, as with all the strategies suggested in this book, the successes and problems should be reviewed as the process develops. This should be modified as appropriate and redesigned where necessary. The key concept through all of this is the learning that comes through experimentation. That is where we as the managers and leaders of health systems have not done well. We have failed to seek out the lessons to be learned and the new territory to be explored. Such exploration *can* be accomplished without risk of capsizing the supertanker and with minimal exposure, financially or perceptually. It does, however, require a willingness to try something new and embrace the precepts as well as the products that have proven successful in other venues and other sectors of American enterprise.

7. Evaluate Progress and Adjust Accordingly

As with all these initiatives, the importance of post-implementation evaluation and ongoing assessment cannot be underscored enough. It is especially relevant in this case, as these ventures are probably the most atypical or pioneering of the group presented in this book.

SUMMARY OF THE STEPS TO TAKING ECONOMIC
ADVANTAGE OF RETAIL AND VISUAL TRAFFIC

- Assign organizational accountability for retail and visual traffic.
- Assemble a team or committee on the retail initiative.
- Test the concept among many audiences.
- Launch with a program involving low commitment, high probability of success.
- Look for partnerships for visual traffic.

- Use the Internet as a prototype.
- Evaluate progress and adjust accordingly.

My prediction is that we will see considerably more activity in this arena in the next two years. Hospitals in Italy are now starting to allow advertising in their hallways; this follows a two-year-old law that prohibited it (Fridoni 2001). In this country it is more an issue of culture than legality that keeps hospitals from pursuing this opportunity, but that is likely to change.

For instance, in April 2001 the Sara Lee Corporation announced that it was giving $5 million to the Forsyth Medical Center Foundation to expand the hospital's center for women's health in Winston-Salem, North Carolina. The executive vice president for Sara Lee noted, "We're proud to put our name on the door and our stake in the ground for better women's healthcare" (Johnson 2001).

Lessons are to be learned from each strategy that will benefit future initiatives and avoid serious pitfalls going forward. Additionally, some valuable lessons will be learned from these endeavors that can be applied to the other initiatives the hospital or health system may be undertaking.

Through it all, the notion of tapping into retail and visual traffic will likely move the organization toward more of a customer-focused, market-oriented entity—and that is a good thing. The common theme throughout this book is to pattern our own organizations after our corporate cousins in other sectors.

REFERENCES

Eridoni, T. 2001. "Italian Hospitals Put Law Allowing Ads on Premises Up to Public Scrutiny." *Wall Street Journal*, May 8.

Johnson, M. 2001. "Sara Lee Gives Money for Women's Center." *Winston-Salem Journal*, April 20.

Conclusion

Two roads diverged in a wood and I—
I took the road less traveled by,
And that has made all the difference.

—Robert Frost

THIS BOOK HAS presented seven strategies that offer potential for just about any healthcare organization in the nation. Individually, these strategies are not likely to radically alter the economic picture of the sponsoring organizations. Collectively, they could represent a fairly impressive arsenal for increasing market share and improving financial performance.

VALUE BEYOND INCREASED SHARE AND IMPROVED INCOME

Perhaps more important than the immediate result from a strategy or a group of strategies is the discipline required and the perspective gained by simply marching down the path. Taking the road less traveled often provides insight into the rest of the organization, as well as perspective on how best to manage the existing operation—that which is already well underway. So it is with these initiatives. By making a commitment to pursue one, two, or more of these strategies, the organization is—by design rather than by default—compelled to develop business plans. In addition, the organization should organize teams, conduct consumer market research, survey other critical audiences, communicate success, and conduct post-implementation assessment—just to mention a few of the common steps for each of these ventures. This exercise alone will be illuminating for some who are not accustomed to this kind of methodical and calculated analysis and confirming for those who are.

PREPARATION FOR RISING CONSUMERISM

Fundamentally, the pursuit of any or all of these strategies has the potential to open up a new vista, provide a fresh perspective, and instill the kind of market-oriented discipline that is engrained in consumer-driven industries throughout the world. As healthcare embraces increasing degrees of consumerism, the type of process described for these strategies will assist the organization in making the transition. Even if healthcare does not become as consumer driven as many experts are predicting, the very exercise of getting closer to customers can only help. An old maxim says "no one ever died from working too hard" (try *that* line on a teenager these days). Along that vein, one could say "no business ever went belly-up by knowing its customers too well."

THE VALUE AND VIRTUE OF VENTURING OUT

Consider the value of good ideas that spring out of new service development and new business exploration. As one highly respected veteran healthcare CEO liked to tell his staff regarding expenses for conventions and symposiums, "If just one of you gets just one good idea from a conference, then the time and resources required to send you are well worth it." So it is with the pursuit of these strategies. If just one really sound concept emerges from the process of ideation, evaluation, substantiation, and incorporation, it has proven worth the effort.

In closing, I would suggest considering the wise and wonderful words of one of America's greatest writers, who gave us all a lesson on venturing out and taking a few risks. Mark Twain observed, "Twenty years from now you will not likely be as saddened by the things you did, as much as by what you didn't do." This is indeed good counsel for just about anybody at just about any time—especially for those of us in the healthcare industry.

About the Author

E. Preston Gee is a widely known writer on healthcare issues and trends. *7 Strategies to Improve Your Bottom Line* is the author's seventh professional book. Other books he has authored include *Columbia/HCA: Healthcare on Overdrive; The For-Profit Healthcare Revolution;* and *Product Line Management: Organizing for Profitability.* In addition to his books, Gee has written more than 40 articles in leading industry publications, ranging from *Modern Healthcare* to the *Journal of Healthcare Management.*

Gee is a senior vice president of strategic planning for the St. David's HealthCare Partnership in Austin, Texas and has held executive management positions in healthcare for more than 15 years. He currently is a member of the board of directors for Texas Hospital Association/Healthshare, and serves on the State of Texas Medicaid Managed Care Committee. He is a past recipient of *Modern Healthcare*'s Up and Comers Award (1994) and received the Quaker Oats Chairman's Team Award for Excellence for new product development. Gee received his M.B.A. and B.S. from Brigham Young University.